The Visual Guide to

Asperger's Syndrome: Meltdowns and Shutdowns

by Alis Rowe

Also by Alis Rowe

The Girl with the Curly Hair - Asperger's and Me
978-0-9562693-2-4

What I have Learned about Life
978-1-9999822-7-0

Website:
www.thegirlwiththecurlyhair.co.uk

Social Media:
www.facebook.com/thegirlwiththecurlyhair
www.twitter.com/curlyhairedalis

The Visual Guide to

Asperger's Syndrome: Meltdowns and Shutdowns

by Alis Rowe

Lonely Mind Books
London

Copyrighted Material

Published by
Lonely Mind Books
London

Copyright © Alis Rowe 2013

First edition 2013
Second edition 2018
Third edition 2020

All rights reserved. No part of this publication may be reproduced in any material form (including photocopying or storing it in any medium by electronic means and whether or not transiently or incidentally to some other use of this publication) without written permission of the copyright owner except in accordance with the provisions of the Copyright, Designs and Patents Act 1988 or under the terms of a licence issued by the Copyright Licensing Agency Ltd, 90 Tottenham Court Road, London, England W1T 4LP. Applications for the copyright owner's written permission to reproduce any part of this publication should be addressed to the publisher.

Warning: The doing of an unauthorised act in relation to a copyright work may result in both a civil claim for damages and criminal prosecution.

For people on the autism spectrum
and the people around them

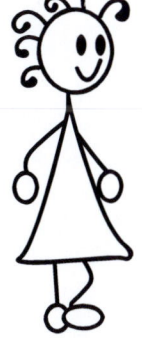

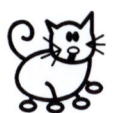

hello

I'll be honest and say that I don't consider meltdowns and shutdowns to be my area of expertise (other than I experience them), nor are they amongst my favourite aspects of autism to write about! They are however, very important to understand as they are a very common and debilitating part of living with autism.

In this book, I describe what meltdowns and shutdowns are, why they might occur, some of the things autistic people can do to help themselves, and what loved ones can do to help them.

I hope you find this book helpful!

Alis aka The Girl with the Curly Hair

Contents

p11   **Overload**

p19   **Understanding 'input'**
- **p29**   Sensory input
- **p35**   Social input
- **p43**   Self-awareness input
- **p47**   Executive function input
- **p49**   Managing inputs

p59   **Meltdowns**
- **p63**   Before a meltdown
- **p71**   During a meltdown
- **p75**   **After a meltdown**

p87   **Shutdowns**
- **p95**   How to recover after a shutdown
- **p101**   Helping to prevent meltdowns and shutdowns

Overload

It is thought that people on the autistic spectrum experience the world more intensely, using more mental effort than neurotypical people

This can cause a person to feel "overloaded"

Meltdowns and shutdowns are typical responses to the feeling of being overloaded

Many things become overloaded...

A circuit	blows
A boat	sinks
A bridge	collapses
A train	won't stop
A computer	won't start
An autistic person	melts or shuts down

Everybody feels overloaded at times

Autistic people however, might experience their feelings of being overloaded a bit differently...

They may feel overloaded by things that neurotypical people hardly notice...

	Reality	Perceived
	●	⬤
	●	●

They may feel overloaded more often...

Level of 'overload' during a typical week for neurotypical versus autistic people

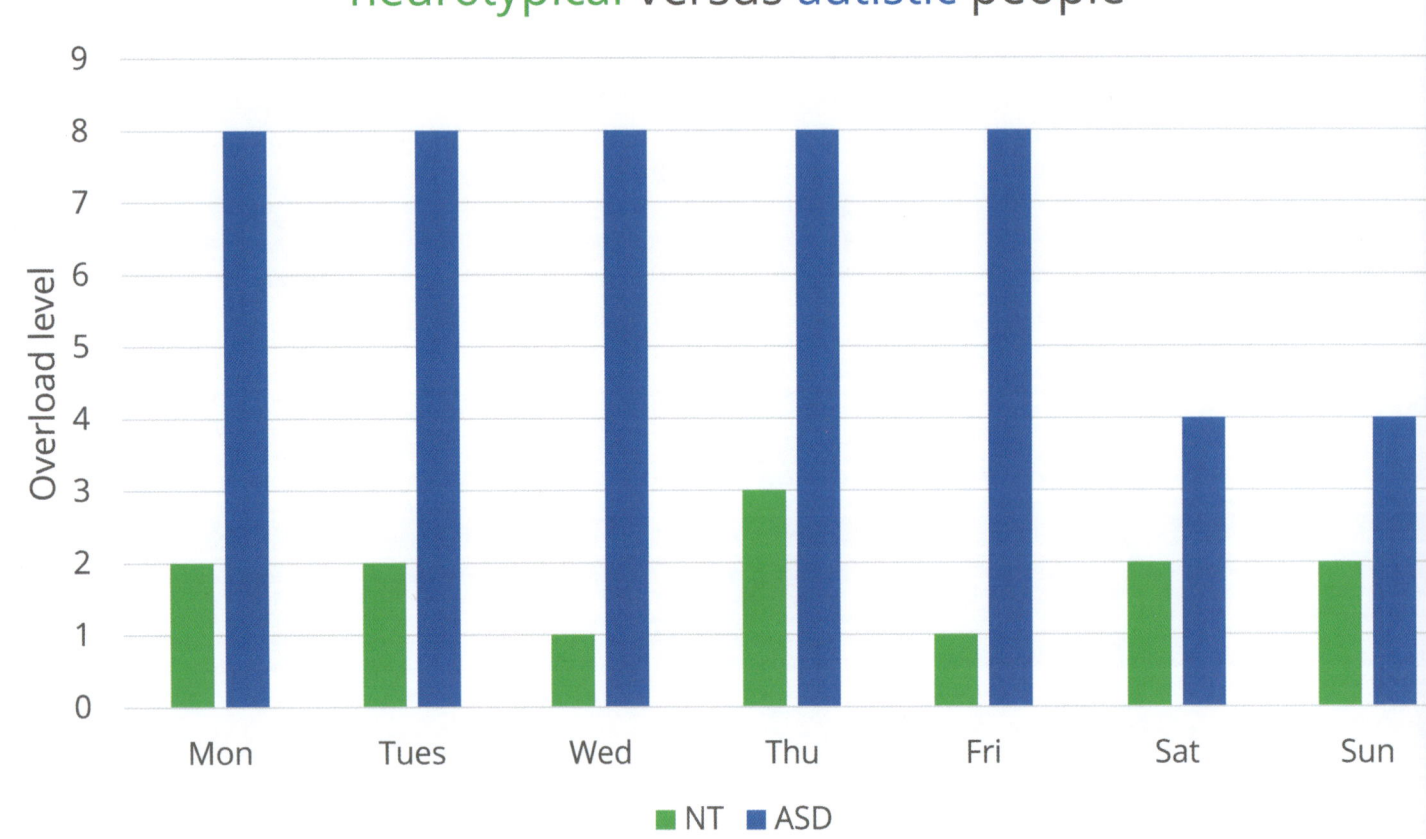

They may experience the feeling of overload more strongly...

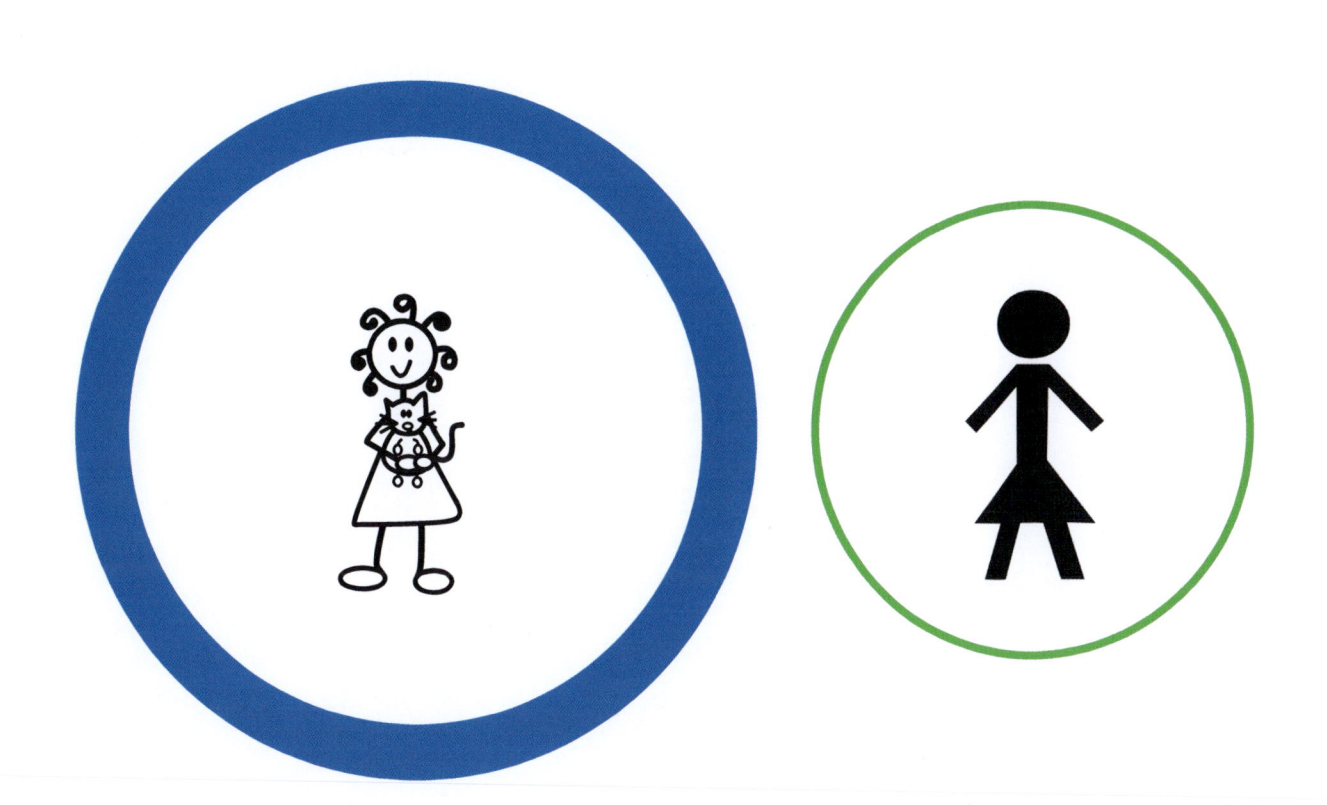

Understanding 'input'

An autistic person's brain is always processing and regulating the information ('input') from the world around them

An autistic person's brain might be unable to process this input properly

An autistic person might feel as though they are having to continually cope with too much input

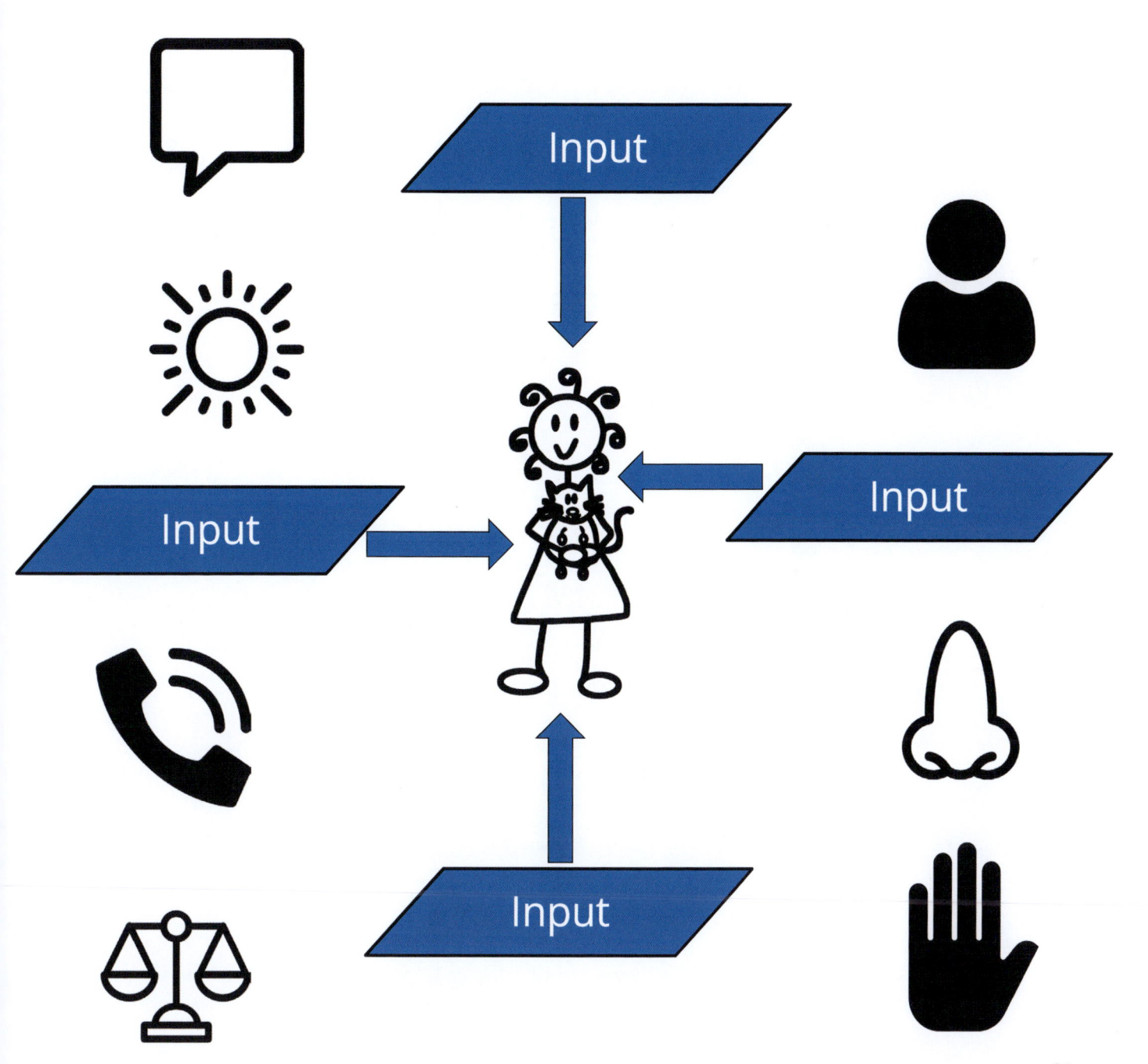

These icons have been designed using resources from Flaticon.com

21

Neurotypical people seem to process this input automatically, whereas for autistic people, it's much more of a manual effort (akin to the effort involved taking the stairs versus an escalator):

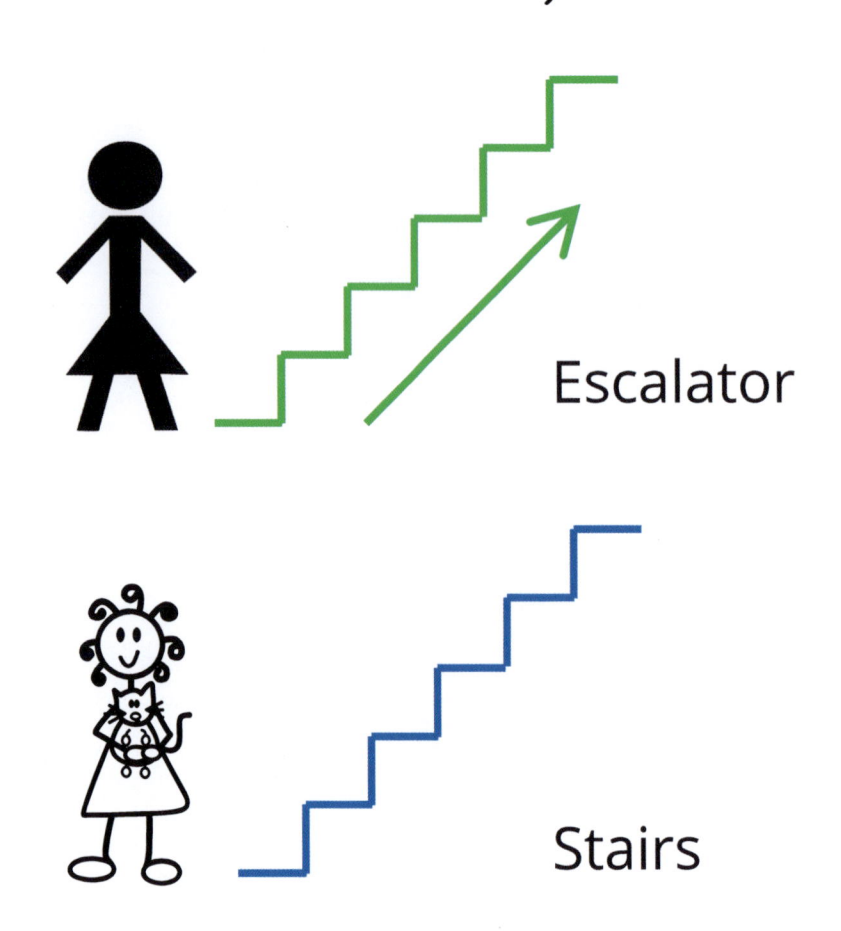

Escalator

Stairs

No wonder autistic people feel exhausted a lot of the time... exhausted in a public environment and exhausted by the time they get home!

The Bucket

A helpful analogy to think about overload is that every autistic person has a 'bucket' and this bucket gets more and more full of input as the day goes on

Without opportunities for the bucket to empty, the bucket will overflow:

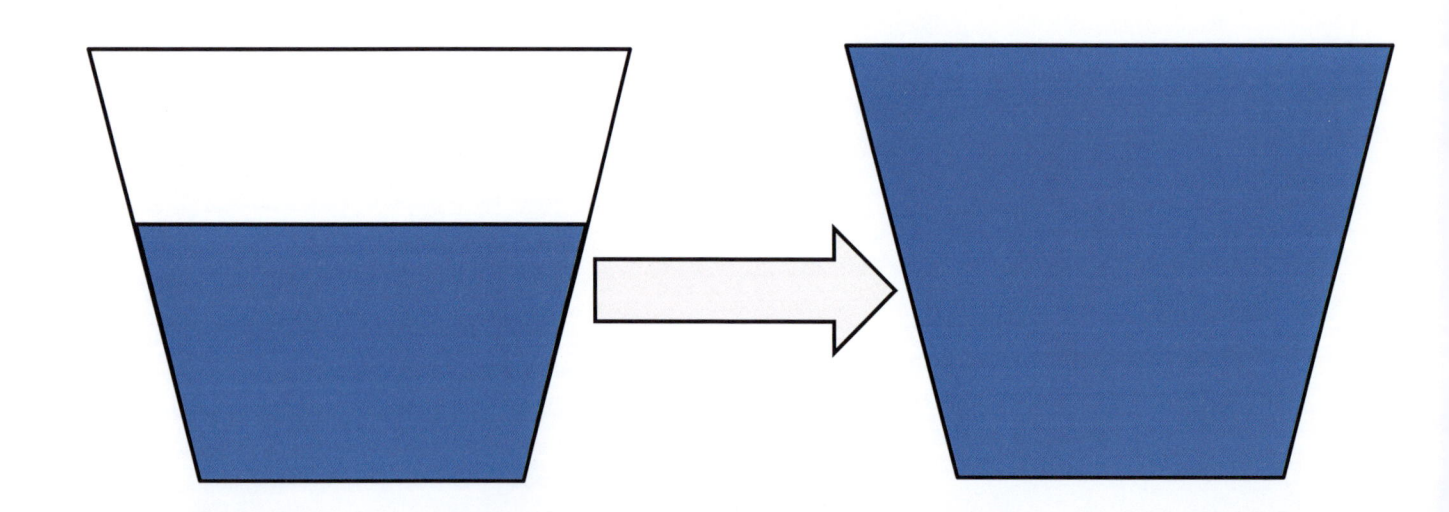

The Filter

Another way of thinking about overload is to consider that a person on the autistic spectrum has difficulty filtering out all the different input in their environment, such as sensory or social information from the person they are talking to

Whereas a neurotypical person can filter out any input that's unimportant, irrelevant or unpleasant, an autistic person might not be able to do so

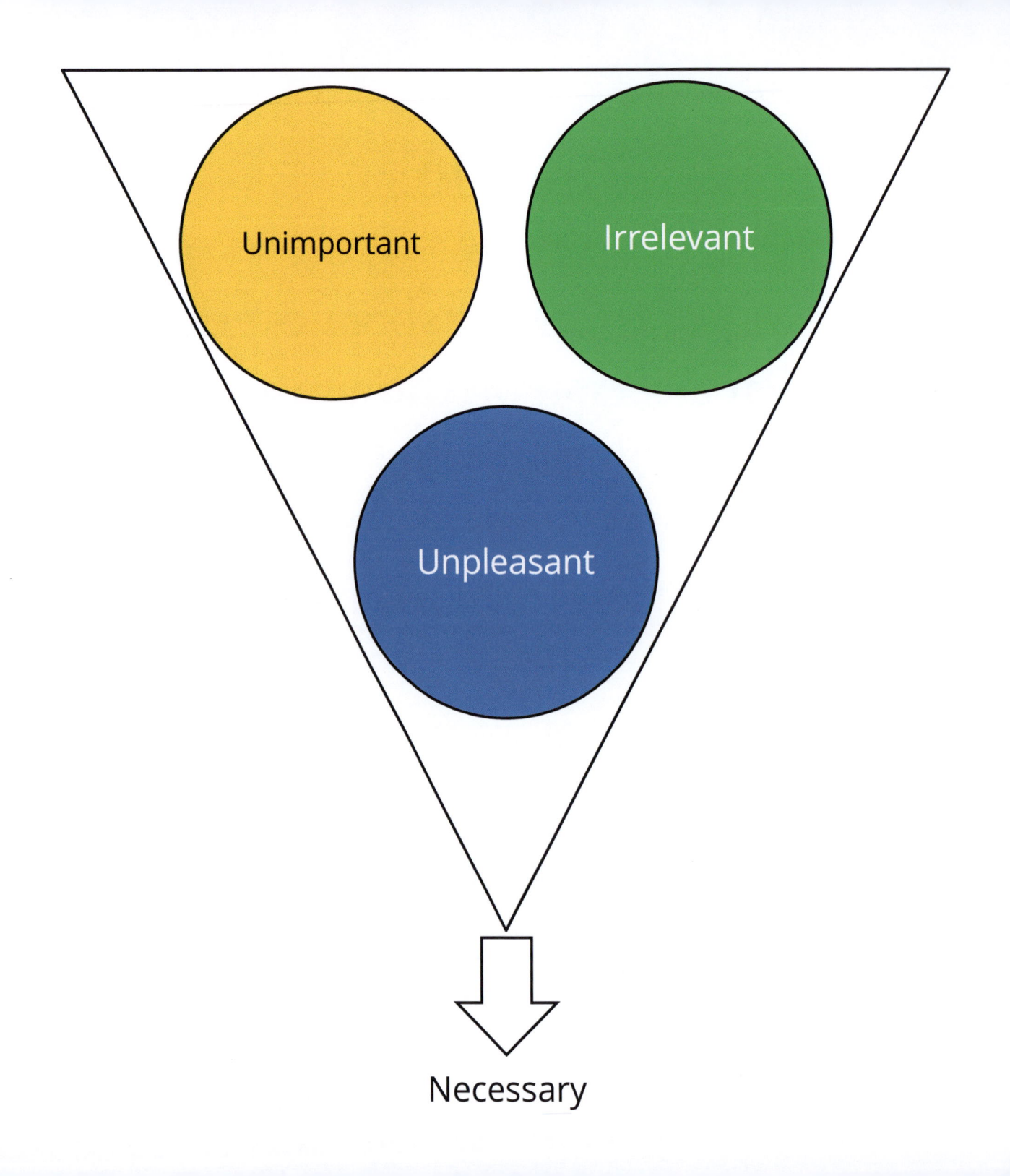

Unimportant

Irrelevant

Unpleasant

↓

Necessary

For example, when The Girl with the Curly Hair meets up with her friend in a cafe for a chat, their experiences are so different...

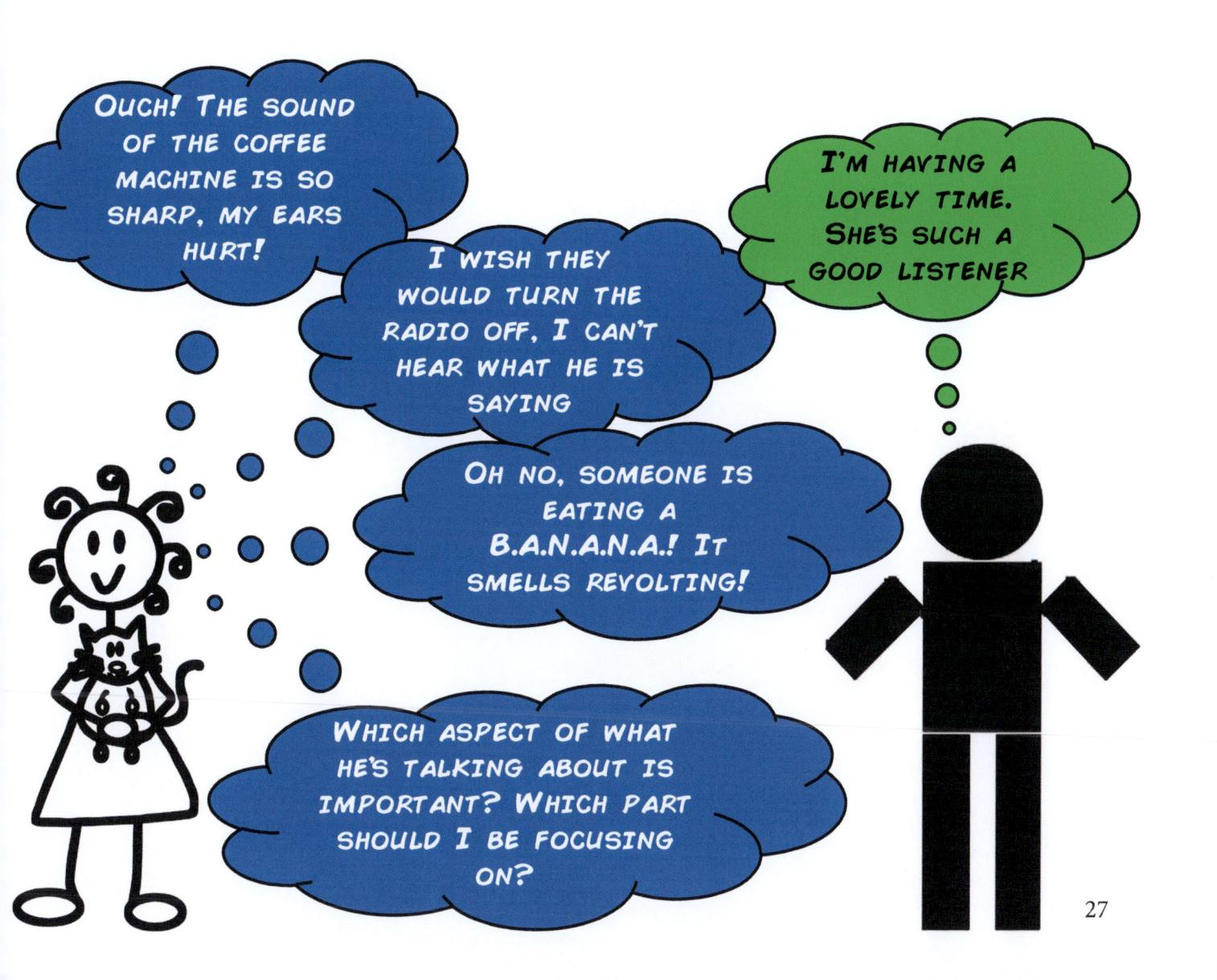

- Ouch! The sound of the coffee machine is so sharp, my ears hurt!
- I wish they would turn the radio off, I can't hear what he is saying
- Oh no, someone is eating a B.A.N.A.N.A.! It smells revolting!
- Which aspect of what he's talking about is important? Which part should I be focusing on?

- I'm having a lovely time. She's such a good listener

Input is *information that is incoming*

Information from this input can be 1) sensory, 2) social, 3) self-awareness and 4) executive function

Sensory input

Sensory input comes from our 5 senses:

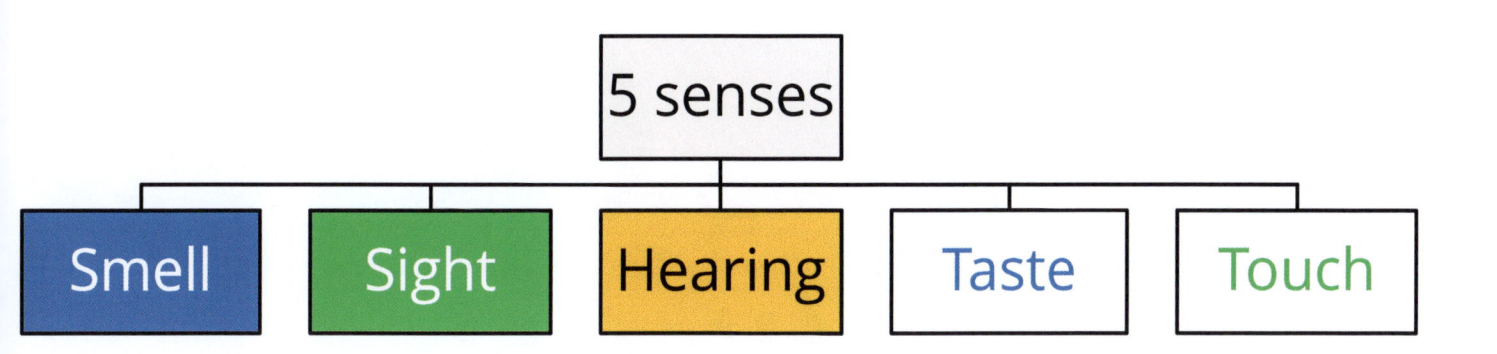

```
                    5 senses
        ┌──────┬───────┼───────┬──────┐
      Smell  Sight  Hearing  Taste  Touch
```

Smell

Strategies that might help autistic people cope with overpowering smells might be:

- I AVOID GOING ANYWHERE WHERE SCENTS MIGHT BE CONCENTRATED. I PREFER SITTING OUTSIDE AT CAFES, FOR EXAMPLE. I LIKE TO SIT NEAR OPEN WINDOWS

- I CHOOSE MY BODY WASH AND SHAMPOO VERY CAREFULLY TO ENSURE I LIKE THE SCENT. SOME PEOPLE MIGHT PREFER COMPLETELY UNSCENTED PRODUCTS

- I CARRY A LITTLE BOTTLE OF LAVENDER OIL. WHEN I SMELL AN UNPLEASANT SMELL, I SMELL MY LAVENDER OIL INSTEAD

- MY FAMILY ARE SENSITIVE TO MY NEEDS AND CONSIDERATE. THEY WON'T EAT STRONG-SMELLING FOODS WHEN I'M IN THE HOUSE

- I ALWAYS ENSURE I HAVE MY OWN 'SMELL-FREE SPACE' AWAY FROM OTHER PEOPLE. THIS IS ESPECIALLY IMPORTANT DURING MEAL TIMES

Sight

Strategies that might help autistic people cope with uncomfortable light might be:

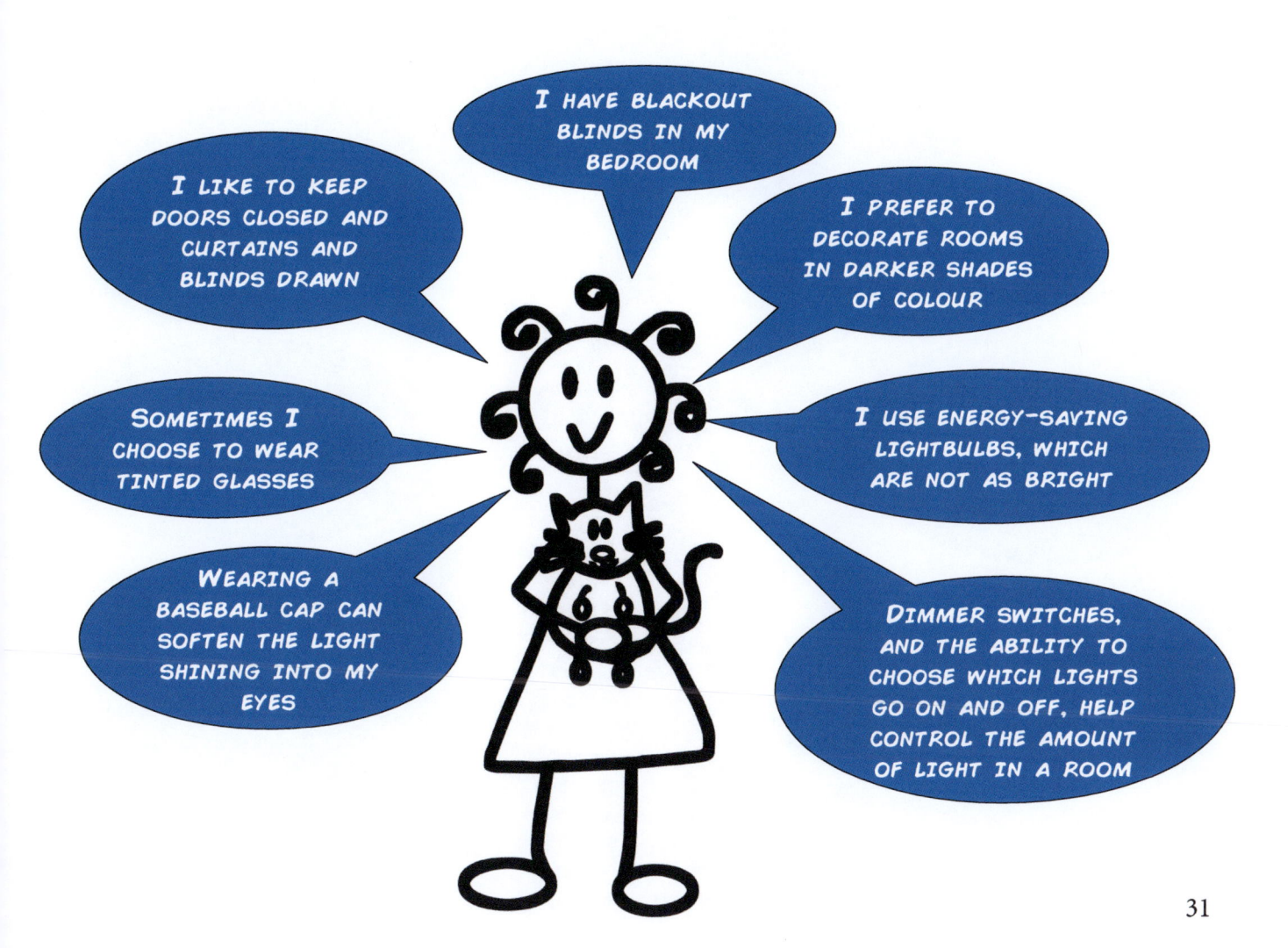

- I have blackout blinds in my bedroom
- I like to keep doors closed and curtains and blinds drawn
- I prefer to decorate rooms in darker shades of colour
- Sometimes I choose to wear tinted glasses
- I use energy-saving lightbulbs, which are not as bright
- Wearing a baseball cap can soften the light shining into my eyes
- Dimmer switches, and the ability to choose which lights go on and off, help control the amount of light in a room

Sound

Strategies that might help autistic people cope with painful noises might be:

- My bedroom is in the quietest part of the house. My office is away from everyone else
- I sleep with a fan on (even when it's cold). The sound of the fan blocks out any outside noise and I find the consistent sound of the fan calming
- I wear noise-reducing earplugs
- I prefer to walk or cycle rather than take public transport which I find very noisy
- I travel during non-peak times when there are less people and less noisy traffic
- I'm not too shy to ask café/restaurant staff if they could turn the radio down. They're usually happy to do this
- I keep windows and doors closed

Touch

Strategies that might help autistic people cope with uncomfortable touch might be:

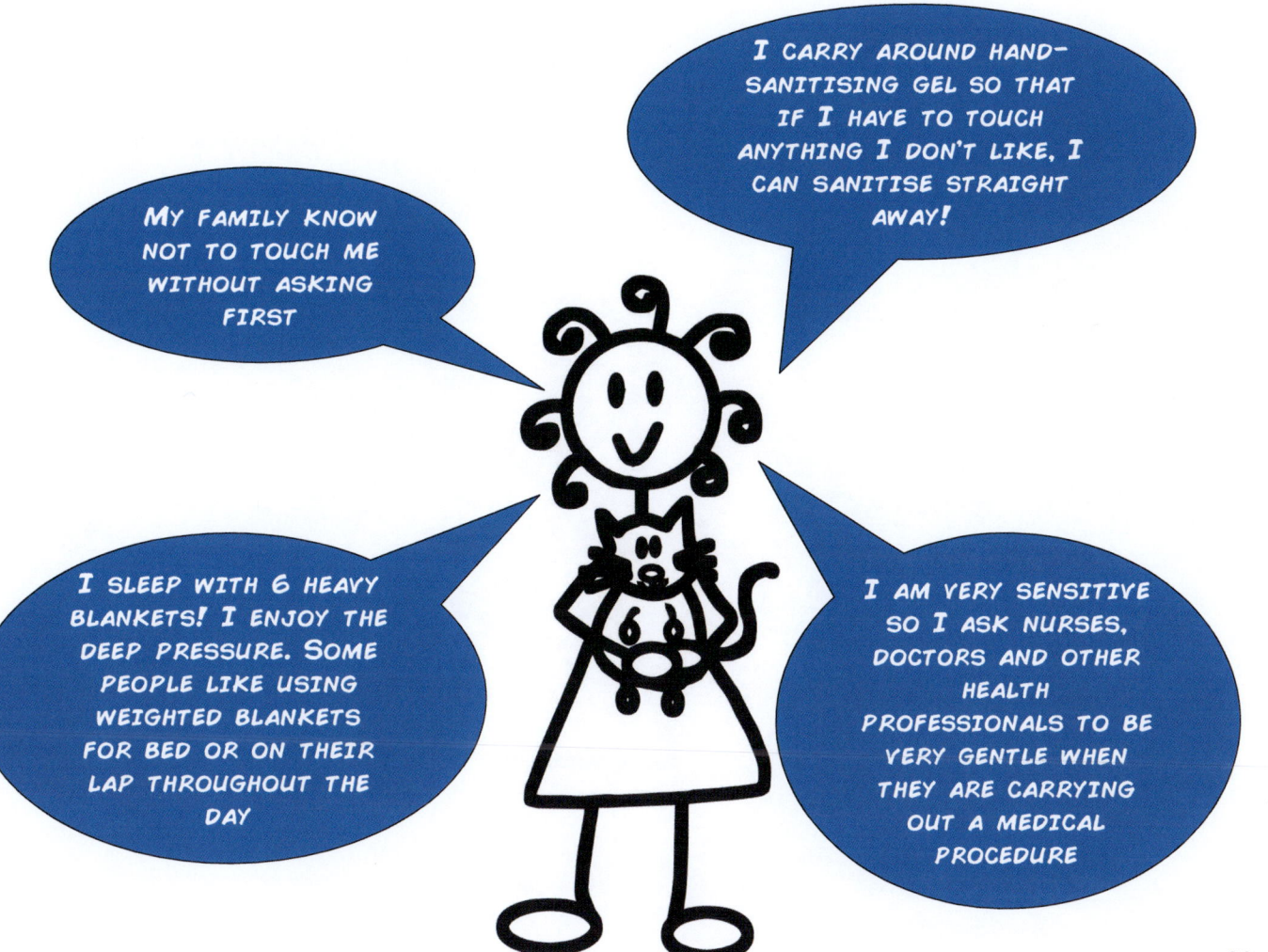

> My family know not to touch me without asking first

> I carry around hand-sanitising gel so that if I have to touch anything I don't like, I can sanitise straight away!

> I sleep with 6 heavy blankets! I enjoy the deep pressure. Some people like using weighted blankets for bed or on their lap throughout the day

> I am very sensitive so I ask nurses, doctors and other health professionals to be very gentle when they are carrying out a medical procedure

Taste

Strategies that might help autistic people cope with overpowering tastes might be:

- There are some foods that I will eat but only when they are prepared in a certain way, e.g. I'll only eat carrots raw and cooked vegetables have to be steamed not boiled or fried

- I like to eat different foods separately. For example, I will eat a plate of vegetables first and then I will have the rest of my dinner afterwards on a different plate

- I try to maintain a healthy diet. I ensure I get the right quantity of food from all the food groups. I try to have a balanced diet

- Consistency is really important to me. I like to have the same foods every day, including the same brands of food

- I prefer mild or bland-tasting foods and I prefer no sauces, spices or oil

Social input

Autistic people have difficulties with social interaction

This means that they don't process and understand 'social input' (body language, words, tone of voice) as automatically as neurotypical people and so social interactions are hard work and confusing

Social interactions can add to the input an autistic person is receiving

Social input can be divided into two main categories:

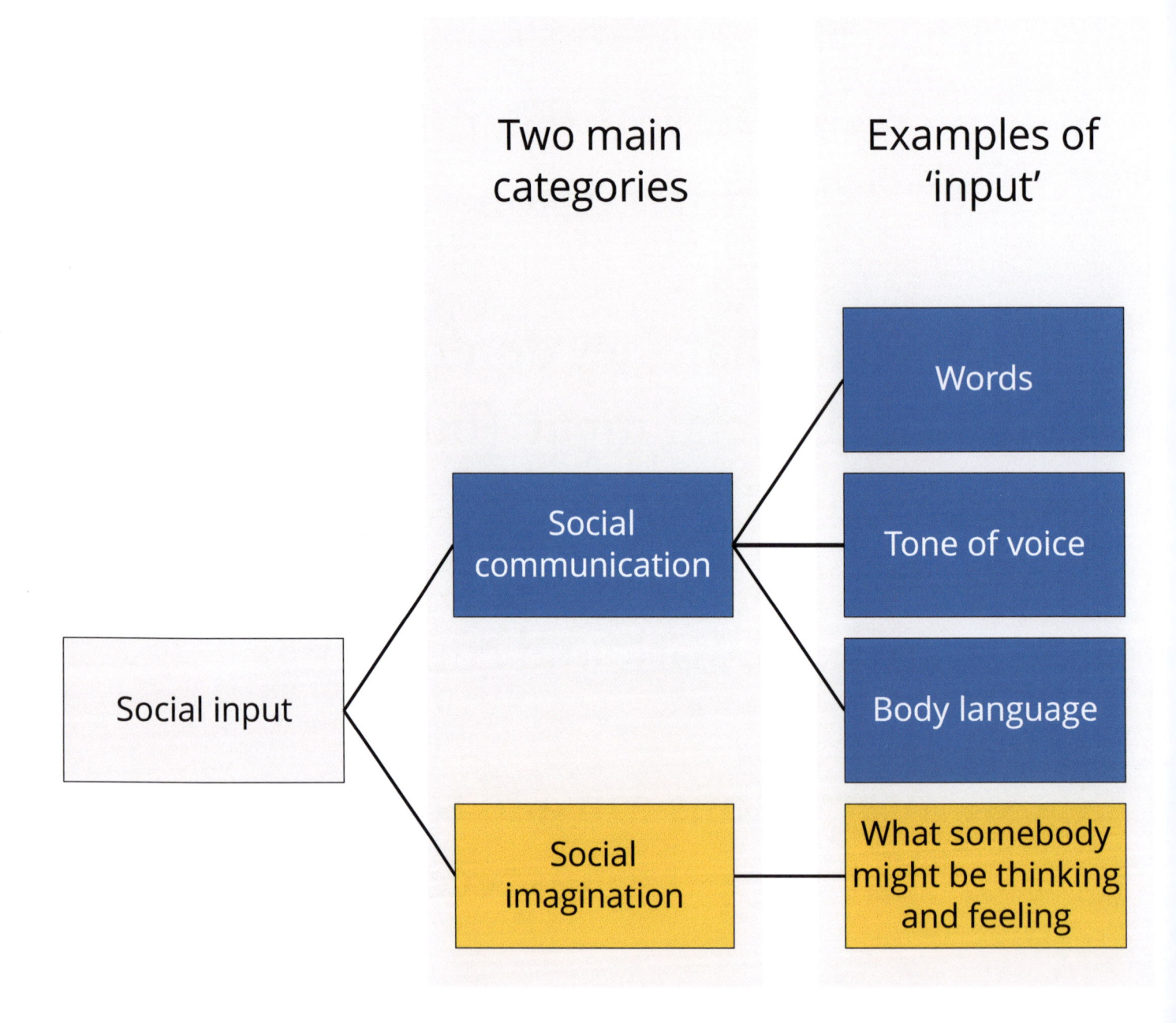

Two main categories	Examples of 'input'
Social communication	Words
	Tone of voice
	Body language
Social imagination	What somebody might be thinking and feeling

Social input
- Social communication
  - Words
  - Tone of voice
  - Body language
- Social imagination
  - What somebody might be thinking and feeling

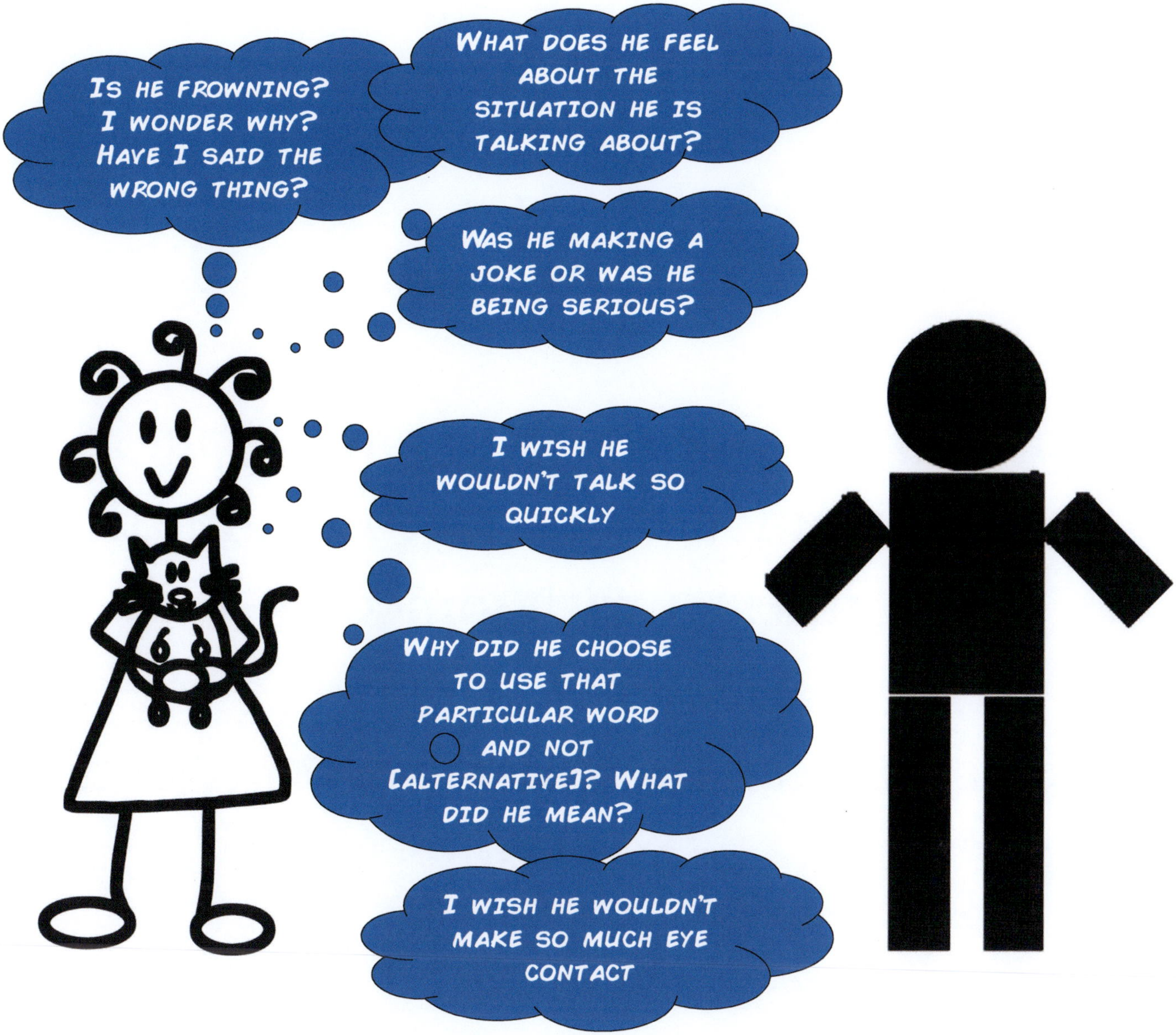
IS HE FROWNING? I WONDER WHY? HAVE I SAID THE WRONG THING?
WHAT DOES HE FEEL ABOUT THE SITUATION HE IS TALKING ABOUT?
WAS HE MAKING A JOKE OR WAS HE BEING SERIOUS?
I WISH HE WOULDN'T TALK SO QUICKLY
WHY DID HE CHOOSE TO USE THAT PARTICULAR WORD AND NOT [ALTERNATIVE]? WHAT DID HE MEAN?
I WISH HE WOULDN'T MAKE SO MUCH EYE CONTACT

Socialising and relating to others is difficult

Autistic people are likely to have to put in an enormous amount of effort any time they interact with someone

Interactions can therefore also contribute to 'overload'

Social Energy Theory

Autistic people might find it helpful to be aware of Social Energy Theory

Social Energy Theory states that everybody has a different capacity for socialising

In general, introverts have less social energy than extroverts

Everyone has a limit for socialising though, which, when reached, is a time when they need to stop and recharge

The social energy tanks look like this when social energy (the amount of energy available for socialising) is at maximum capacity:

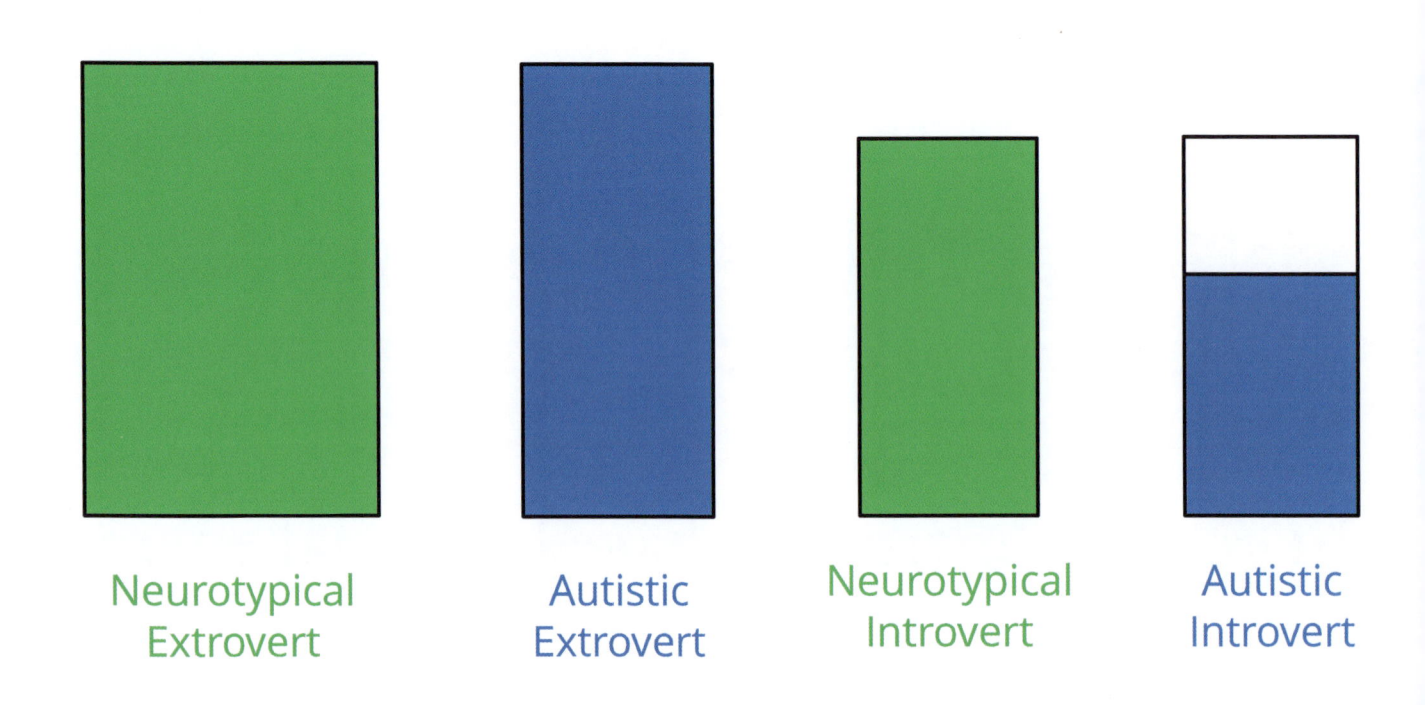

| Neurotypical Extrovert | Autistic Extrovert | Neurotypical Introvert | Autistic Introvert |

The tanks illustrate that autistic people have less capacity for socialising than neurotypical people

It is very important for autistic people to learn how to manage their social energy and to be somewhat in control of the social interactions they have every day or every week

Too many social interactions can contribute to input, and too much input can lead to meltdowns and shutdowns

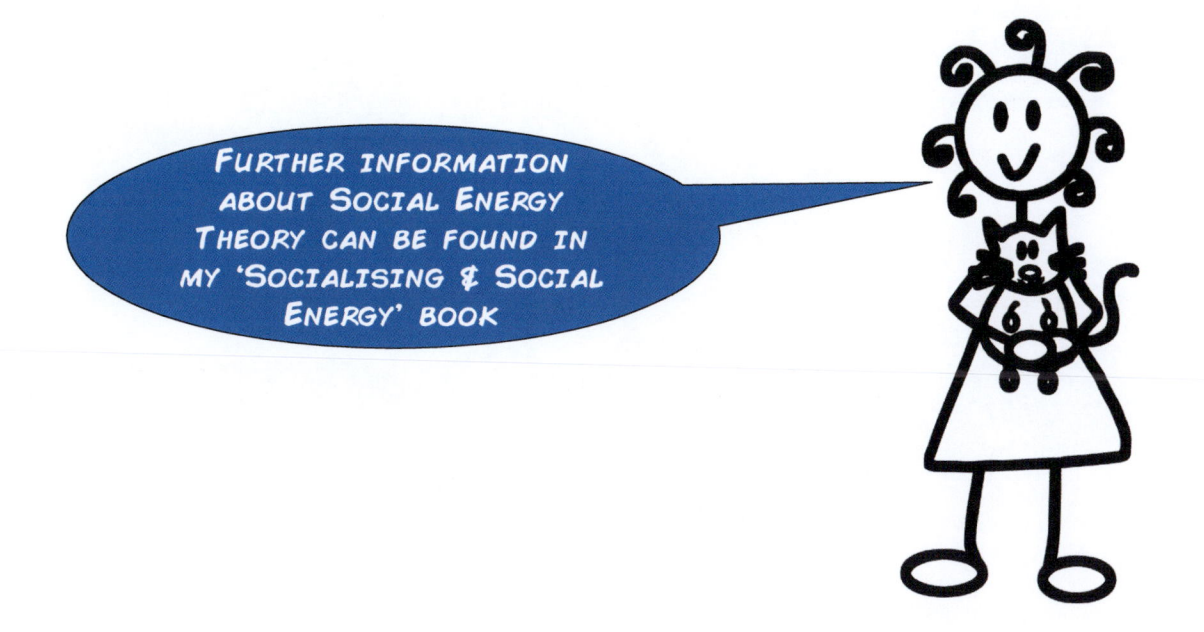

> Further information about Social Energy Theory can be found in my 'Socialising & Social Energy' book

Some strategies that might help autistic people manage their social energy include:

- My family are respectful of my need for space, quiet and time alone. They try not to disturb me
- I tend to leave social occasions early
- I am assertive enough to politely say "no" when people invite me to social occasions I don't feel I have enough energy for
- If I have a day that involves a lot of socialising, I make sure that I recharge the following day
- I spend time with people one on one rather than in groups
- I have plenty of Alone Time throughout the day, every day

Self-awareness input - bodily

This is the information that comes from within our body and sends a message to our brain. The ability to perceive these signals is known as interoception:

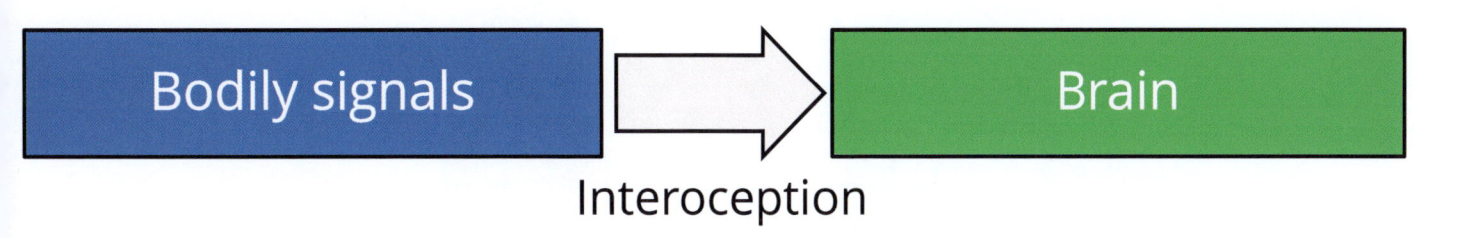

| Bodily signals | → | Brain |

Interoception

For example, a person receives signals of hunger, thirst, exhaustion, feeling cold, or needing to go to the toilet

These signals can contribute to input

An autistic person may have difficulty recognising these signals, or perhaps they can identify them but they don't do anything to rectify the feeling (for example they don't eat when they need to, or they don't put a jumper on when they feel cold)

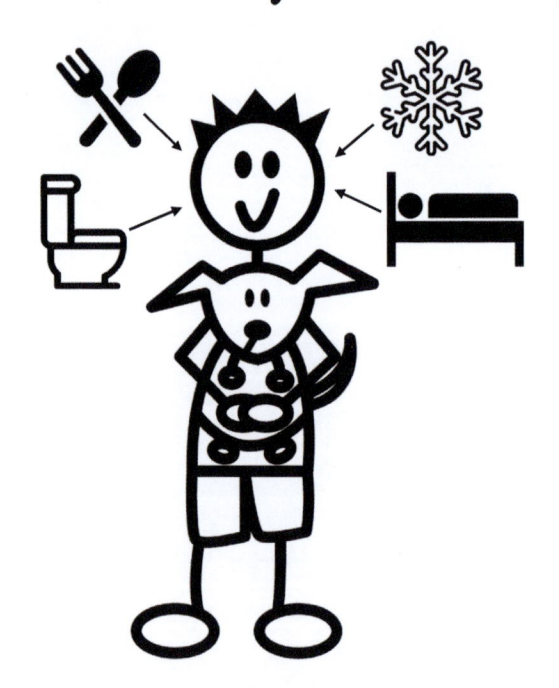

Self-awareness input - thoughts and feelings

Self-awareness input can also be the thoughts and feelings that we have at any given moment

It can include having very strong emotions that are difficult to process

Autistic people may also be prone to giving themselves 'instructions' in order to get through social situations and daily life generally. For example, they might be following 'social scripts'

These thoughts and feelings are inputs as well

For example, here are some thoughts The Girl with the Curly Hair has just before she meets up with her friend...

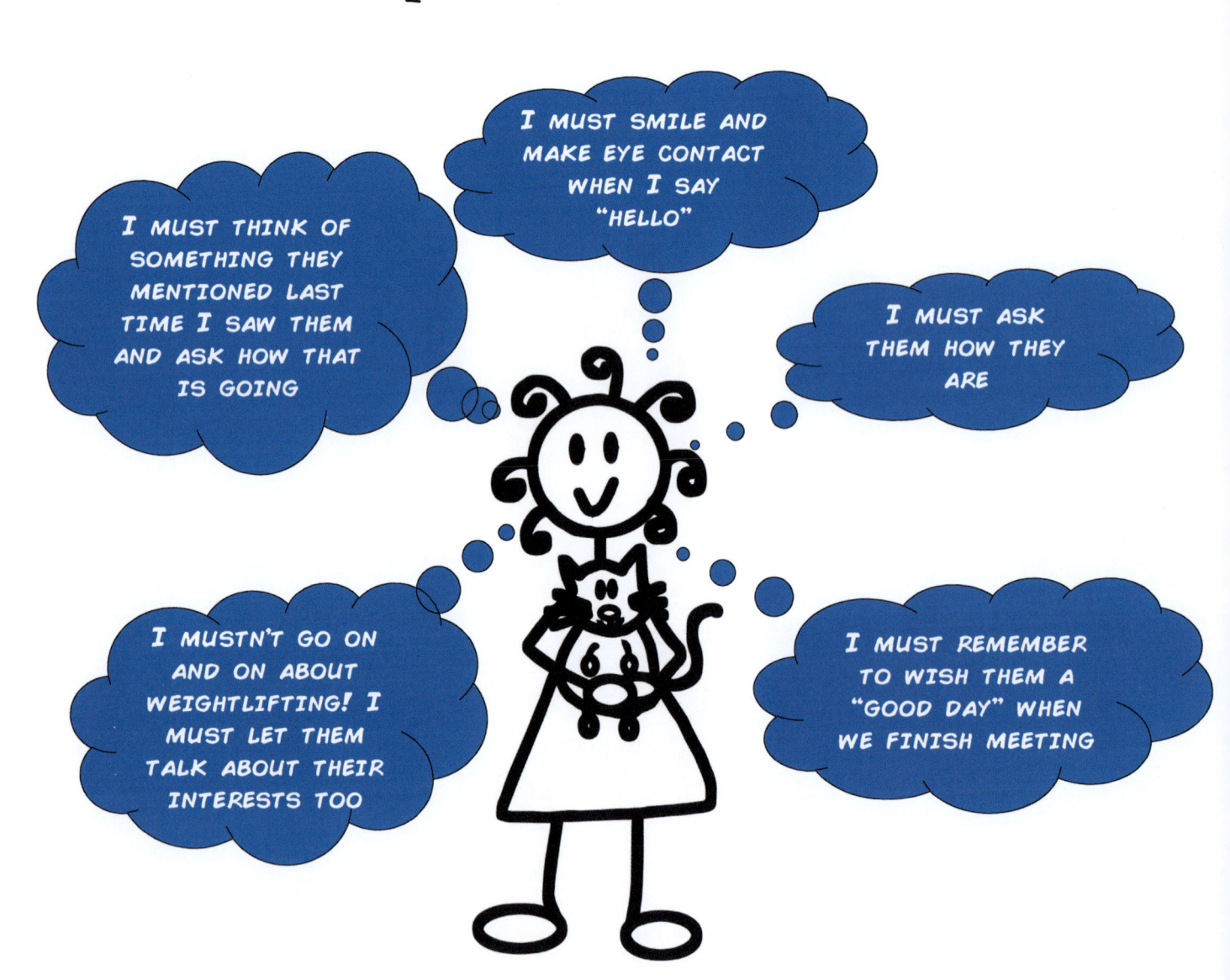

- I must smile and make eye contact when I say "hello"
- I must think of something they mentioned last time I saw them and ask how that is going
- I must ask them how they are
- I mustn't go on and on about weightlifting! I must let them talk about their interests too
- I must remember to wish them a "good day" when we finish meeting

Executive function input

Executive function is the set of mental skills that helps people get things done

It includes skills such as planning, prioritising, sequencing, starting and finishing tasks

Autistic people can greatly struggle with executive function, causing them to feel overloaded

> FURTHER INFORMATION ABOUT EXECUTIVE FUNCTION CAN BE FOUND IN MY 'EXECUTIVE FUNCTION' BOOK

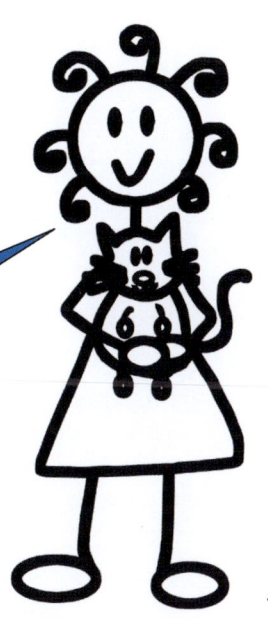

Managing inputs

If a person continually receives input throughout the day everyday, it can cause them to feel exhausted

Autistic people probably receive input more consciously than neurotypical people. Many autistic people are very sensitive and notice and absorb all sorts of data, sensations and feelings that neurotypical people do not notice. Autistic people have a higher level of *input sensitivity*

Imagine sensitivity as a gauge. Autistic people perhaps have a higher level of sensitivity to input than neurotypical people

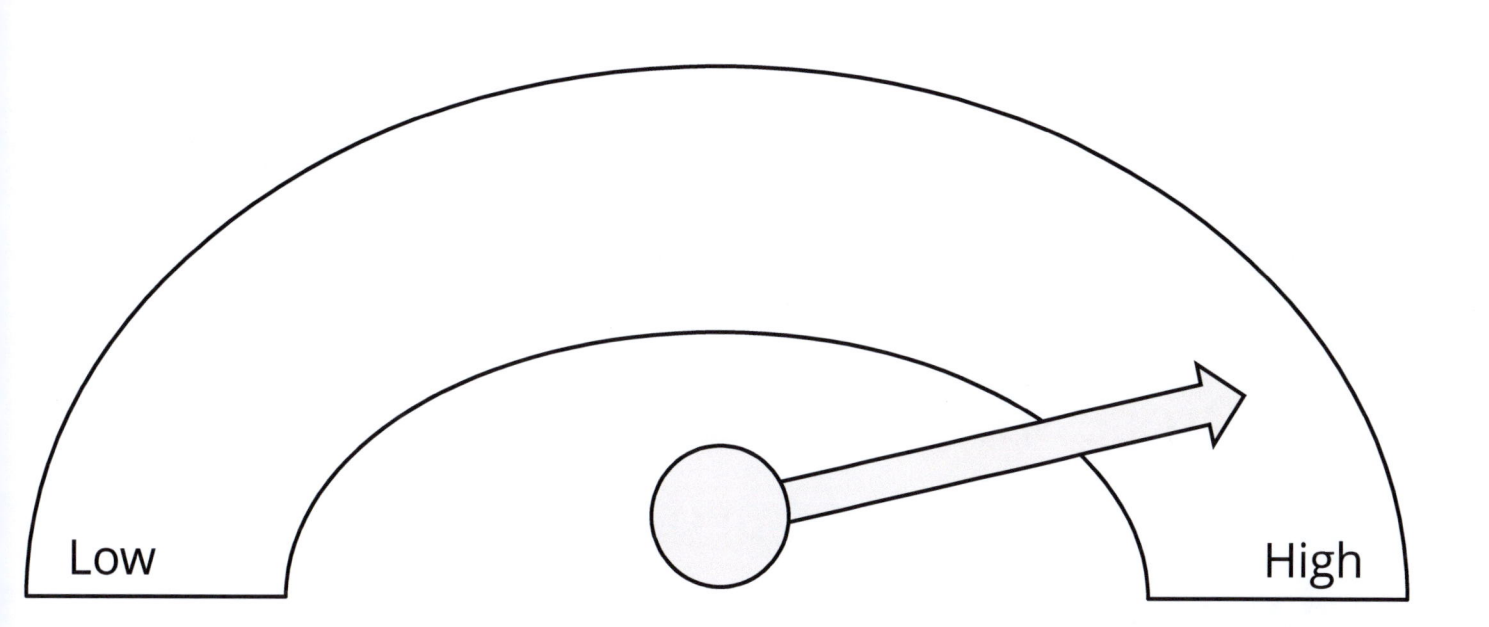

Low

High

Autistic people are also more likely to have difficulty *processing* the input. Neurotypical people seem to process input with ease and more automatically. Autistic people have a lower level of *input processing*

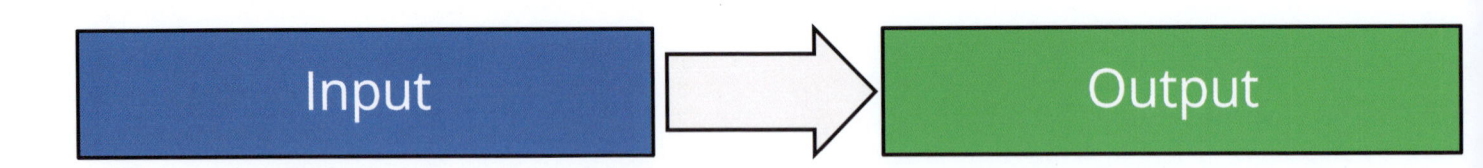

| Input | → | Output |

'Processing' should be a simple in-out procedure. Autistic people perhaps struggle with this processing more than neurotypical people

Input can be managed in a couple of ways:

1) It can be offset with output

This is applicable when the input is sensory- or bodily-related. For example, a person can try to counteract a loud noise by wearing noise-reducing earplugs. A person can have a glass of water when they feel thirsty

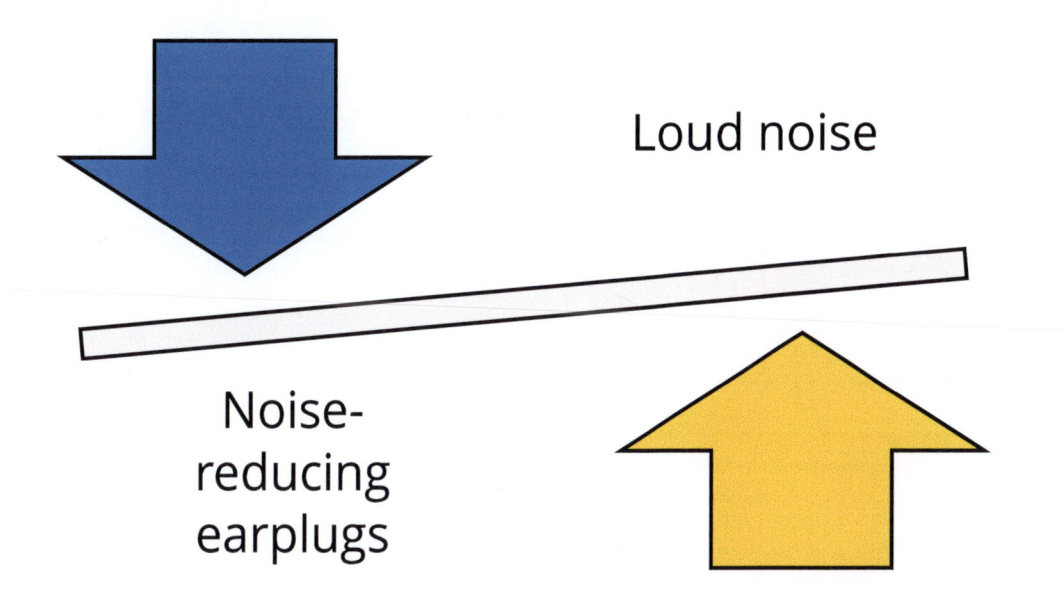

Loud noise

Noise-reducing earplugs

2) Regular breaks or 'Recharge Time' throughout the day

An autistic person is likely to need time throughout the day on their own or in a quiet place where there is no input. This means that their capacity for receiving input is deliberately restricted

For example, if a person were in a busy environment and socialising all day then they would be receiving input all day:

Graph to show how input can accumulate throughout the day if no breaks are taken

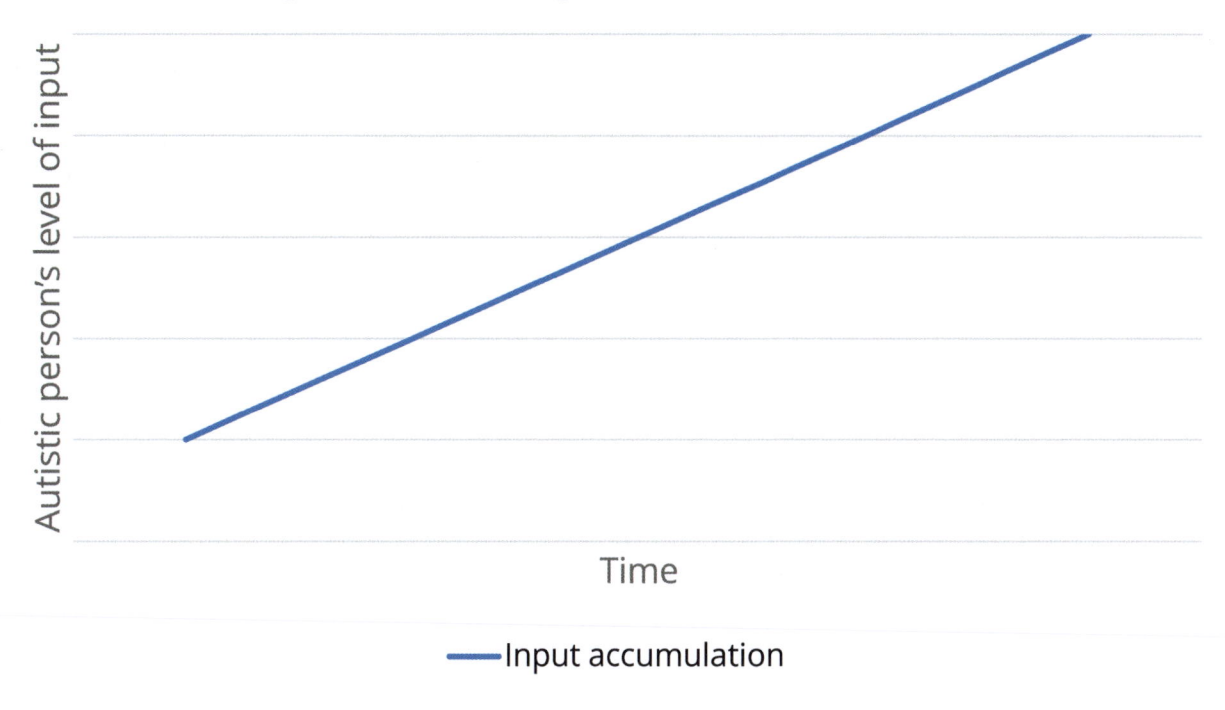

Y-axis: Autistic person's level of input
X-axis: Time
— Input accumulation

Total input exposed to: High

If they took a few breaks during the day, there would be times when they were not receiving input. Therefore, at the end of the day the total amount of input they had been exposed to would be less:

Graph to show how input might accumulate throughout the day if regular breaks were taken

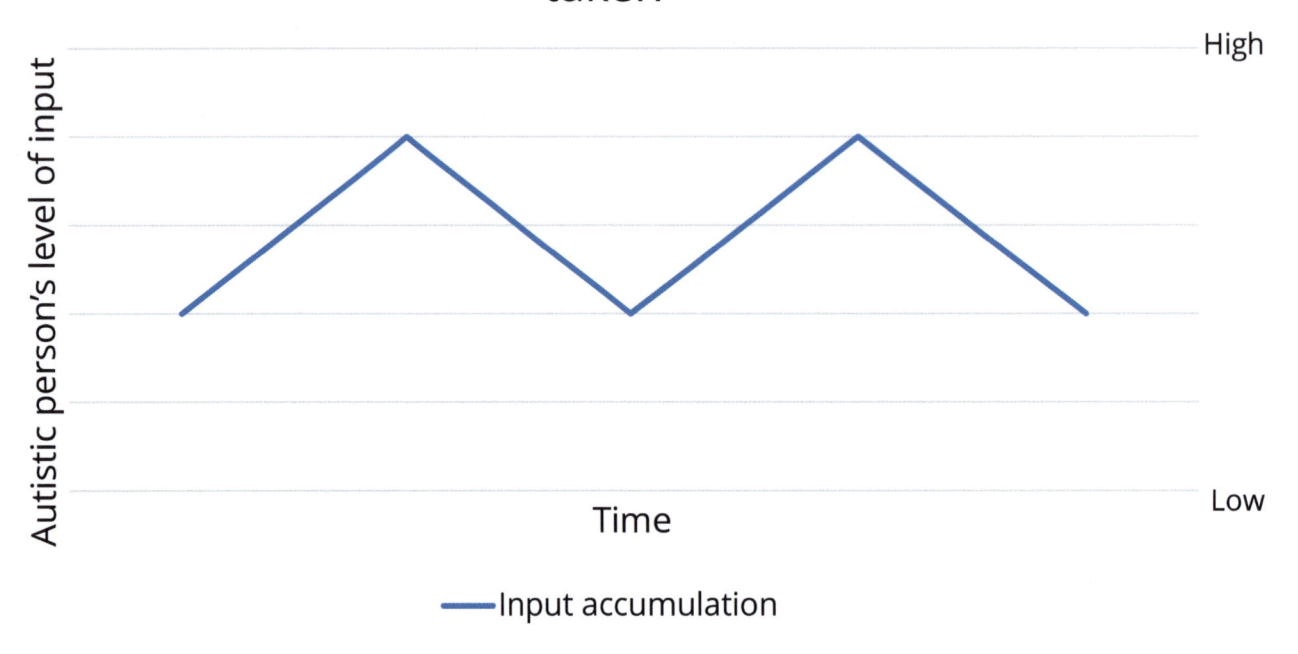

Y-axis: Autistic person's level of input (High to Low)
X-axis: Time
— Input accumulation

Total input exposed to: Much lower

Recharge Time will be different for different people. For example, some people will feel recharged by being on their own, others will feel recharged by going for a walk, others will feel recharged by listening to music. When a person has a chance to recharge, it means the input level they receive has a chance to decrease

Autistic people will likely greatly benefit from learning to successfully reduce and manage the amount of input they are exposed to. It will help them to have more energy, to feel less stressed, and may even reduce the chances of meltdowns and shutdowns from happening

Summary of inputs

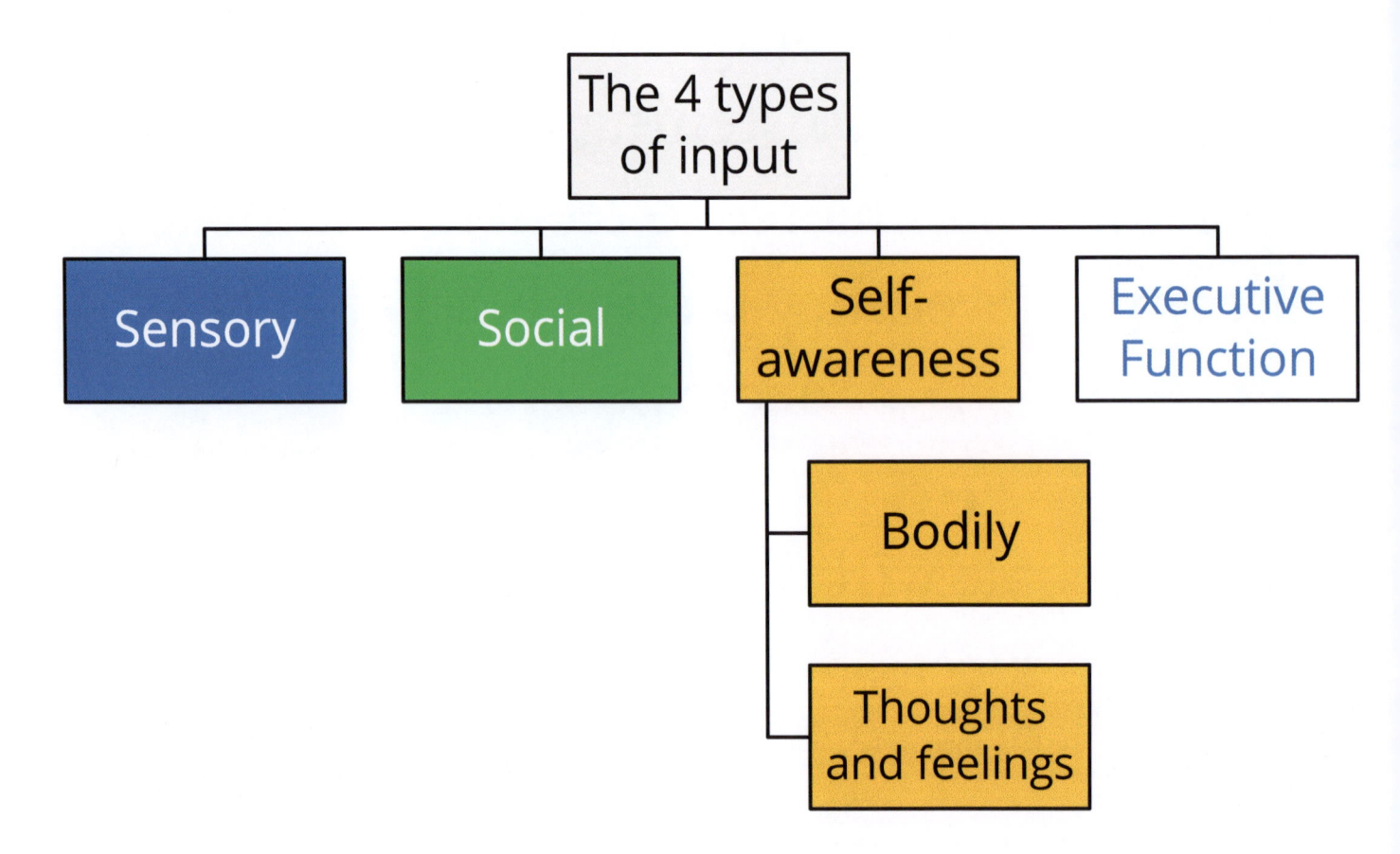

- The 4 types of input
  - Sensory
  - Social
  - Self-awareness
    - Bodily
    - Thoughts and feelings
  - Executive Function

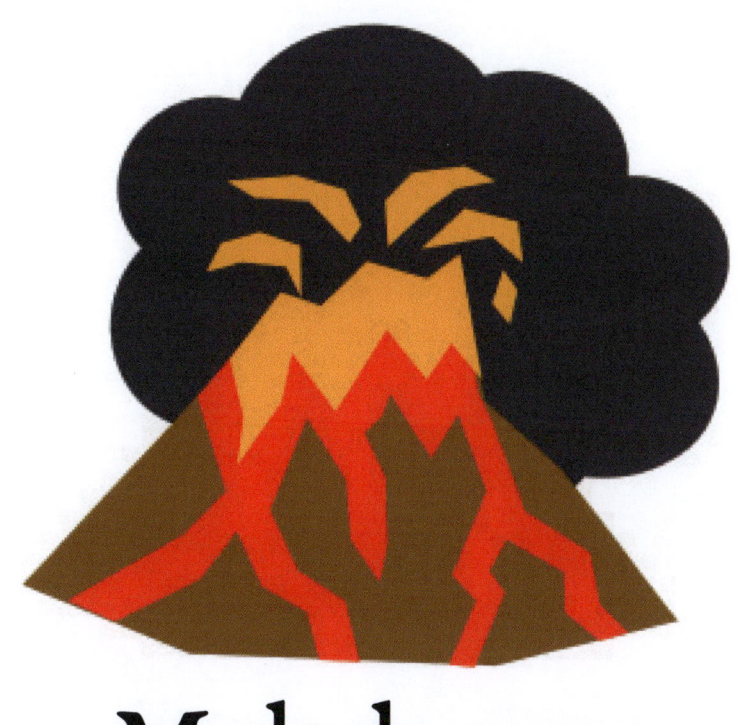

Meltdowns

How does The Boy with the Spiky Hair describe meltdowns?

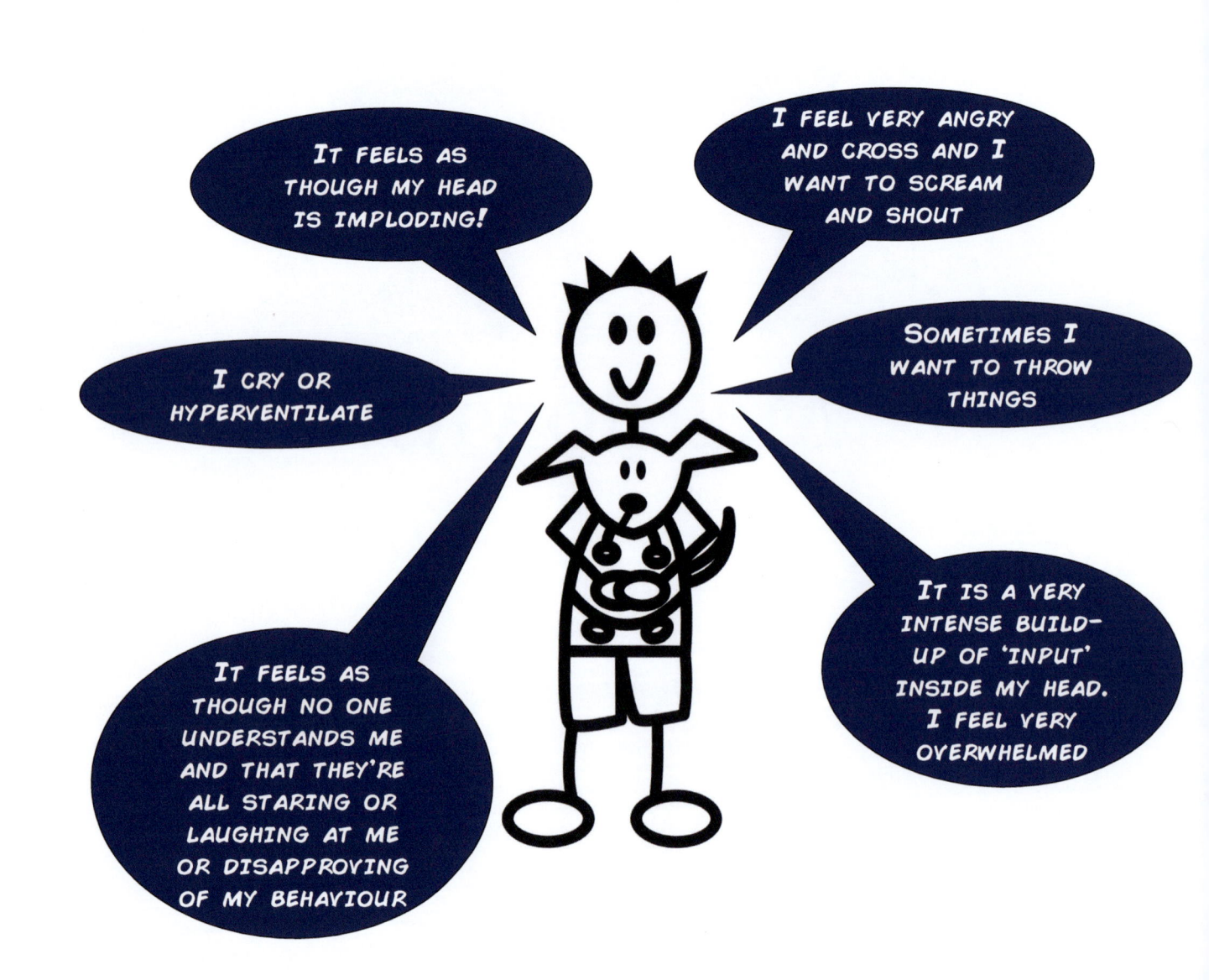

- It feels as though my head is imploding!
- I feel very angry and cross and I want to scream and shout
- I cry or hyperventilate
- Sometimes I want to throw things
- It feels as though no one understands me and that they're all staring or laughing at me or disapproving of my behaviour
- It is a very intense build-up of 'input' inside my head. I feel very overwhelmed

The Girl with the Curly Hair says...

> When I'm about to have a meltdown, there is a tiny part of my mind that says, very logically, "Stop right now" and "You have a choice now about what is going to happen next"...

> ...But another, much bigger, part of my mind either ignores this or even sort of answers back and says "I don't care!" and then the meltdown just happens

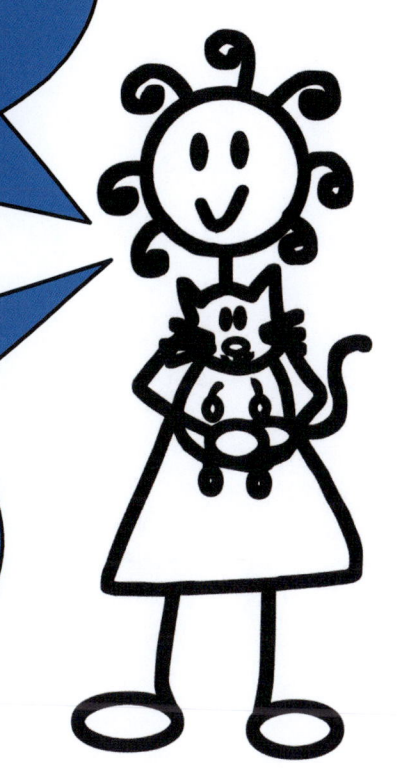

Meltdowns may seem similar to tantrums but there are some significant differences:

Tantrum
- Driven by a want or a goal
- They check you are paying attention
- They act this way only when they have an audience
- Once they have got what they want, the behaviour stops

Both
- Hitting
- Kicking
- Shouting
- Crying
- Throwing things

Meltdown
- Is a reaction to feeling overstimulated
- They do not care if they get your attention
- Their behaviour will continue, even without an audience
- The behaviour will only end once they have calmed down. There is nothing they "want" so there is no goal

Before a meltdown

Here are some strategies that might help autistic people recognise when a meltdown might happen:

Think about the bigger picture

- What else has happened that day or that week? Has it been particularly stressful of overwhelming?
- What is going on around you right now? What is the current environment like? Is it busy or stimulating?
- When did you last eat or drink? When did you last go to the toilet? Do you feel physically comfortable, such as the right temperature?
- Remember that a meltdown does not always occur because of one particular trigger, it can be a combination of factors

Look out for any signs

- What do you/does your loved one do when they are feeling overwhelmed? Do you/they start talking a lot? Do they go very quiet? Do they start fidgeting? Do they look physically uncomfortable?

Try to stop the meltdown before it happens

- The person could take a break in quiet or on their own
- The person could tend to their physical needs, such as eating a meal
- The person could do something they find relaxing
- The person could use something to block out the input they are receiving, such as earplugs or closing their eyes, or they could use a type of input that they find calming such as a weighted blanket
- The person could direct their feelings towards something more constructive, such as ripping up paper, throwing ice cubes in the bath, bouncing a ball, or jumping on a trampoline. It is often important to find an activity that helps release the tension a person feels

An autistic person could themselves try to recognise their own signs and symptoms so that they know when they are beginning to feel overloaded, e.g.

Signs	Symptoms (feelings)
• Talking a lot • Not talking • Sweating • Pacing • Fidgeting • Flapping • Tearful	• Butterflies • Ears feel hot • Sick • Irritable • Cross • Very upset

Then they could learn what to do when they feel this way, before a meltdown happens

Once the autistic person has recognised the signs, make sure they know what they can do to manage the situation, for example:

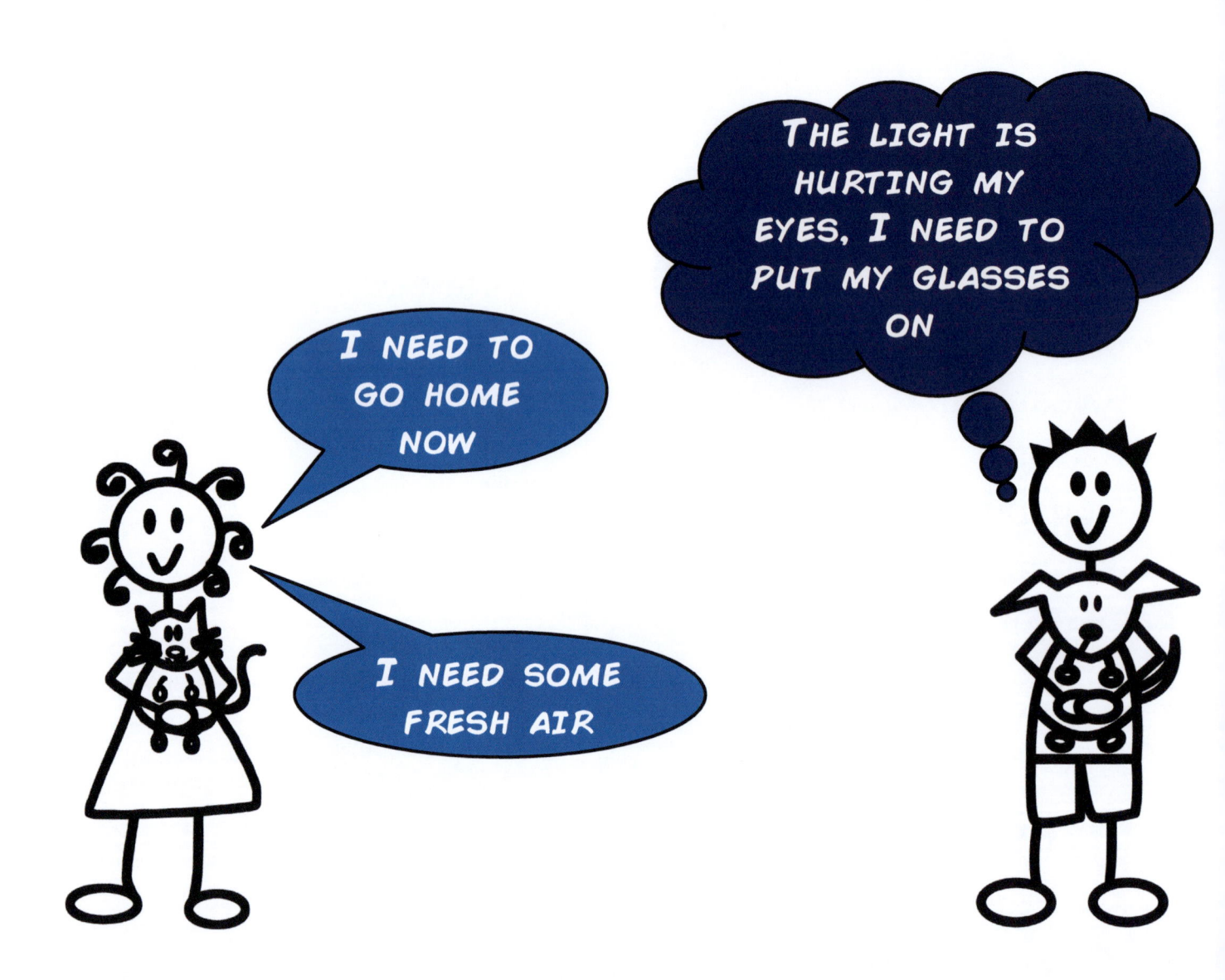

I NEED TO GO HOME NOW

I NEED SOME FRESH AIR

THE LIGHT IS HURTING MY EYES, I NEED TO PUT MY GLASSES ON

One of the most helpful things is to always ensure the autistic person has an 'exit strategy' for the situation they are in:

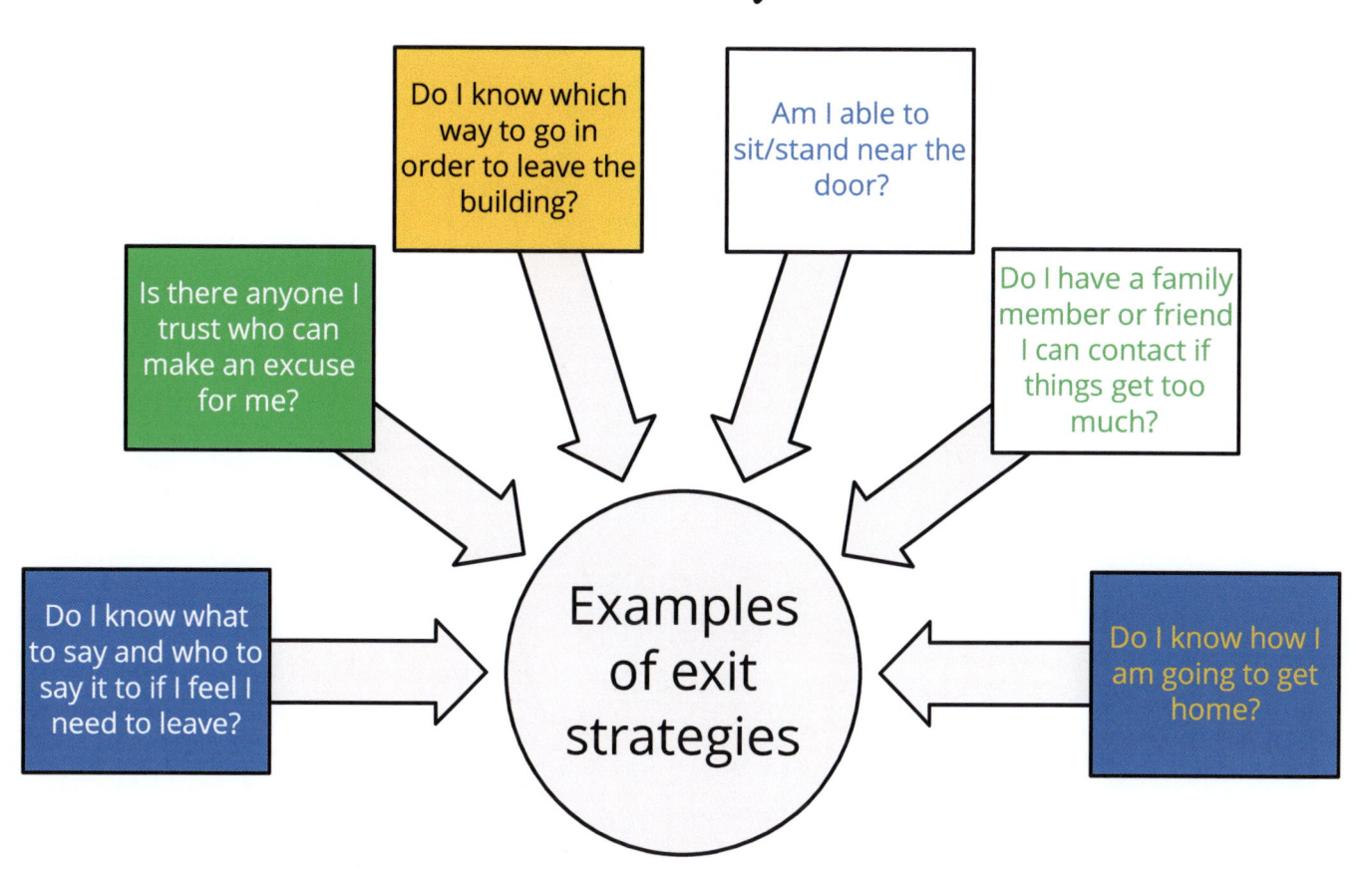

- Do I know which way to go in order to leave the building?
- Am I able to sit/stand near the door?
- Is there anyone I trust who can make an excuse for me?
- Do I have a family member or friend I can contact if things get too much?
- Do I know what to say and who to say it to if I feel I need to leave?
- Do I know how I am going to get home?

Examples of exit strategies

If the autistic person does suddenly want to rush off, try to let other people know that they are safe so that other people do not worry. Once they are home, they could send a message to say they have arrived safely, for example

Calming strategies or leaving the situation quickly enough could actually prevent the meltdown from occurring:

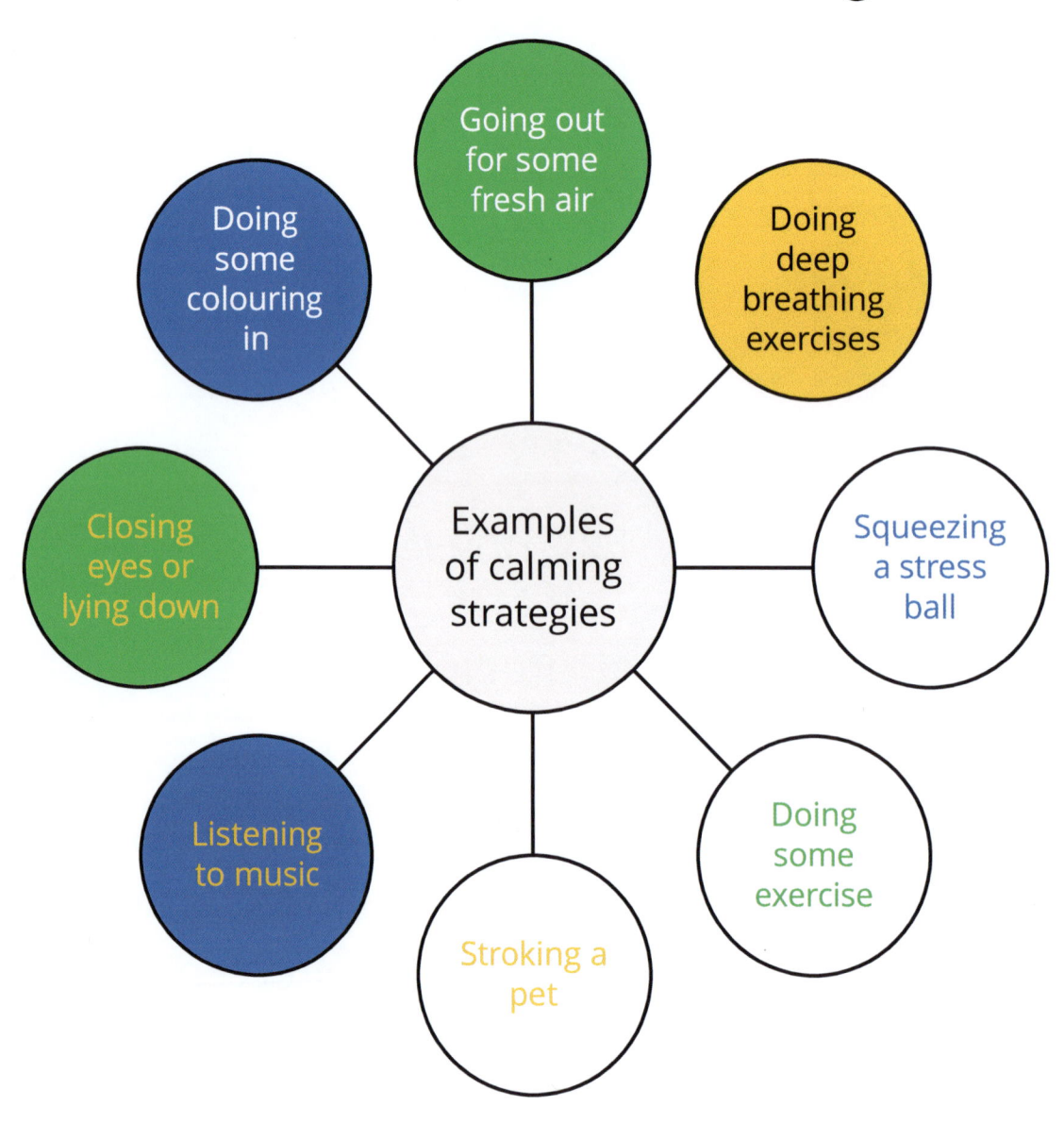

Examples of calming strategies:

- Going out for some fresh air
- Doing deep breathing exercises
- Squeezing a stress ball
- Doing some exercise
- Stroking a pet
- Listening to music
- Closing eyes or lying down
- Doing some colouring in

When a meltdown is coming…	What can I do?
What can I do right now to manage the situation?	•I can ask someone for help •I can take a break from the situation •I can work out what the problem is and try to resolve it myself
Have my physiological needs been met?	•Do I need the toilet? •When did I last eat? Am I hungry? •When did I last drink? Am I thirsty? •When did I last move about? •When did I last have some fresh air?
What can I do to express my discomfort in a safe way?	•I can do some exercise •I can throw ice cubes in the bath •I can tear up a piece of paper •I can ping a rubber band against my skin •I can scream into a pillow •I can hit a punching bag
What can I do that is calming?	•I can stroke my pet •I can listen to relaxing music •I can lie down •I can go outside for some fresh air

The Boy with the Spiky Hair

sometimes becomes aggressive in public. He has learned these 4 techniques that help him control his behaviour:

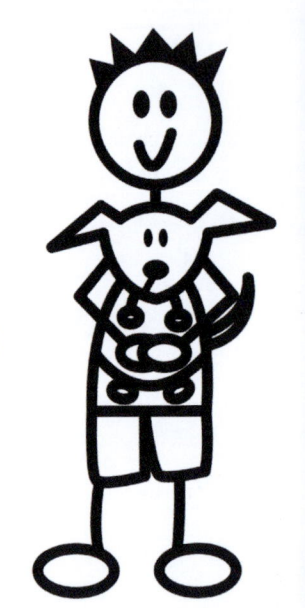

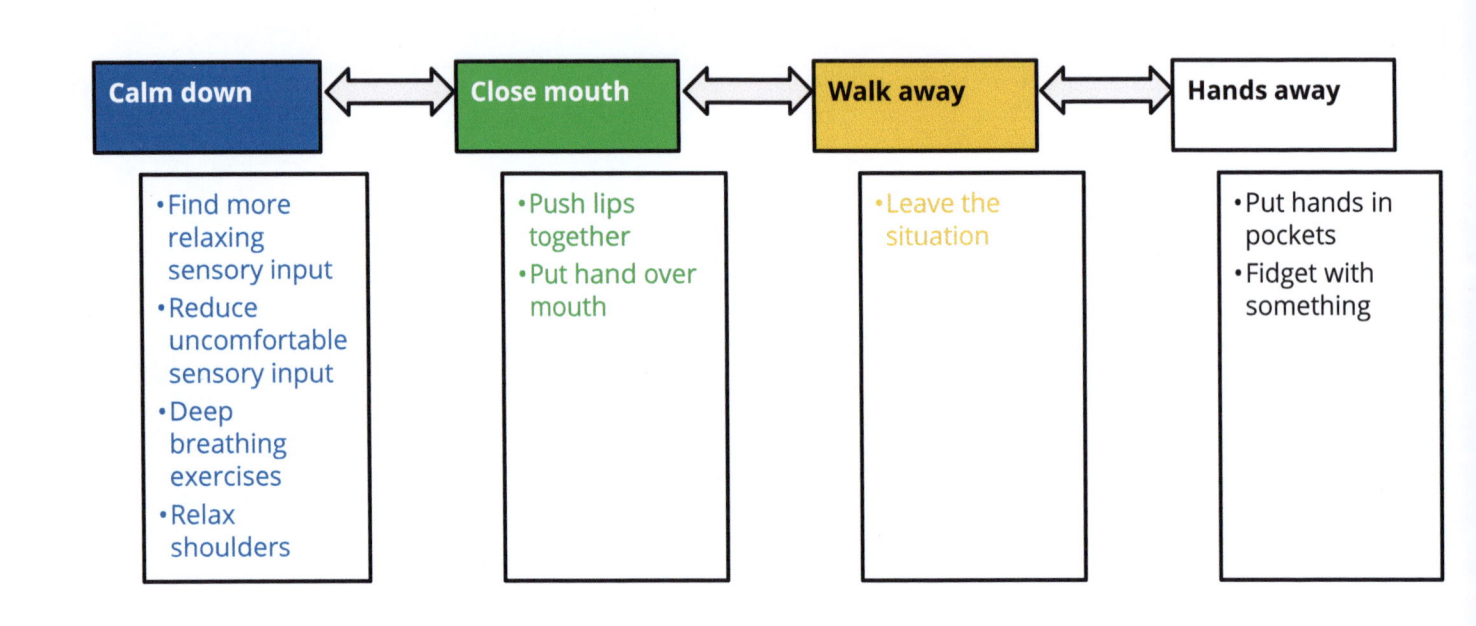

Calm down	↔	Close mouth	↔	Walk away	↔	Hands away
• Find more relaxing sensory input • Reduce uncomfortable sensory input • Deep breathing exercises • Relax shoulders		• Push lips together • Put hand over mouth		• Leave the situation		• Put hands in pockets • Fidget with something

During a meltdown

Here are some suggestions for things a loved one can do as a meltdown is happening:

Make sure they are safe

- If you are out, get them home or take them somewhere private and quiet
- Do not let them wander off in case they hurt themselves (remember, they are most likely feeling out of control at this time)
- Some people like to be held very tightly, others may hate it
- Is there a particular comfort item you can give them?
- Can you give them an alternative for self-harming, e.g. paper to rip up, a pillow to hit, ice cubes to throw in the bath?

Make sure their environment is safe

- Make sure there are no potentially dangerous objects lying around
- Clear away toys they might trip over, remove glass they could cut themselves on, etc.

It's not usually a good idea to attempt to ask the autistic person "what's wrong?" or to ask "How can I help?" during a meltdown

This is the natural thing for many neurotypical people to want to do

Trying to communicate with someone whilst they are having a meltdown is just creating even more input!

It's probably best to talk about the meltdown *after* it has happened

Autistic adults may benefit from figuring out what helps them specifically during meltdowns. In time, they may know how to manage their own meltdowns in the best way. **The Girl with the Curly Hair** for example…

> When I feel myself about to have a meltdown, I just like to go to my room and allow the emotions to come out. I don't want anyone around me, all I want is space. I'll come out when I'm ready

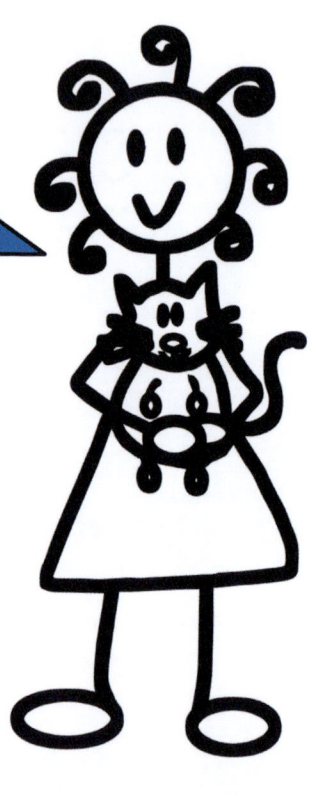

After a meltdown

After a meltdown, an autistic person may experience different feelings, such as:

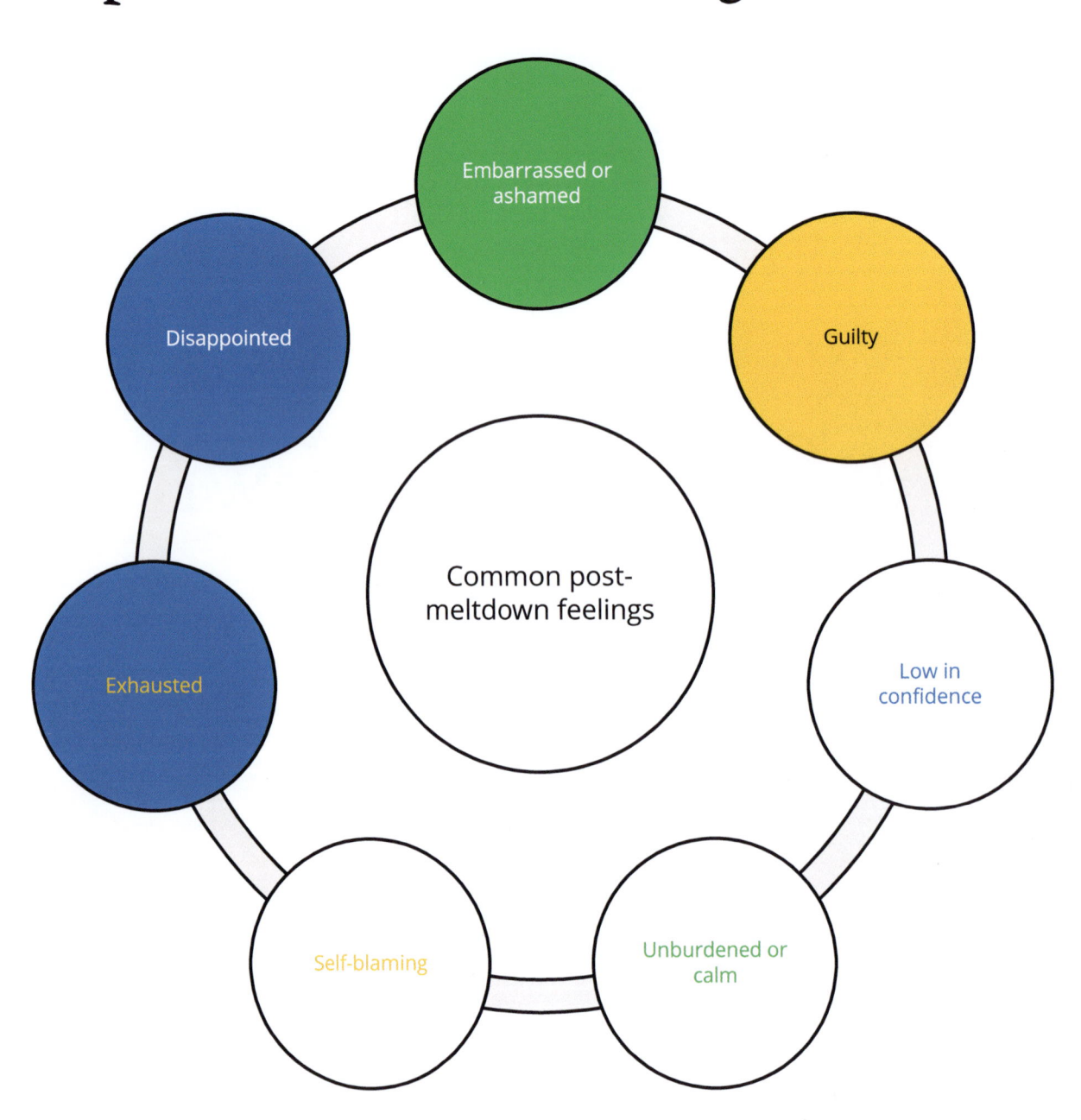

- Embarrassed or ashamed
- Disappointed
- Guilty
- Exhausted
- Low in confidence
- Self-blaming
- Unburdened or calm

Common post-meltdown feelings

Young autistic children may not have the maturity to experience such strong post-meltdown feelings, but **autistic adults** can feel absolutely awful

Remember that it's also much easier for children to 'get away' with difficult behaviour than it is for adults, so adults might feel uncomfortable about the way in which they behaved during their meltdown

Feeling	Reason
Embarrassment	•Meltdowns can be completely out of character – an autistic person can appear very 'normal', pleasant, calm, gentle, quiet and yet has these awful occasional outbursts •Wondering who witnessed the meltdown
Calm and unburdened	•Meltdowns can release a lot of pent up stress •A meltdown might be the only way a person is able to communicate their feelings
Self-blame or disappointment	•Person might feel they ought to be able to control themselves •Person might feel angry that they 'allowed' a meltdown to happen •It might feel like a setback

Feeling	Reason
Guilty	For causing a disturbance to the people around them
Low in confidence	Person might think that other people now think less of them
Exhausted	Person might feel dazed and "zoned out" because meltdowns are exhausting

After a meltdown, I find it helpful to avoid using the word 'should' (for example, "That shouldn't have happened" or "I should have been able to control myself"). That sort of language makes me feel awful

I find it helpful to reflect on what has happened in a constructive way. Were there any signs a meltdown was going to happen? What could (the word 'could' is better than 'should!') I have done differently? What could I change next time to reduce the chance of this happening again?

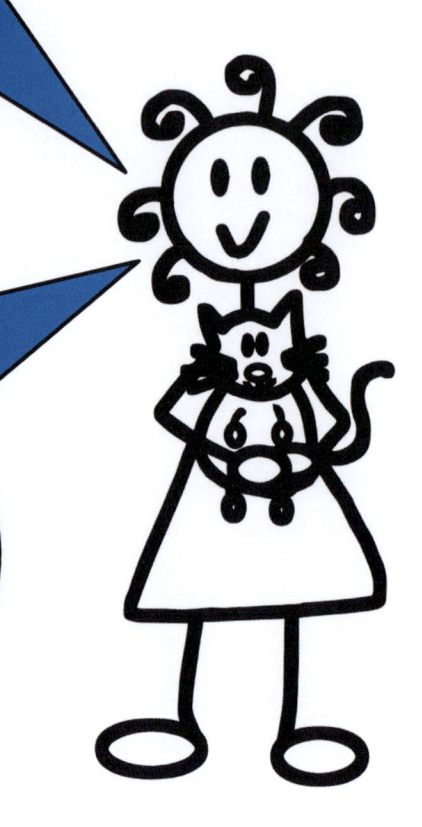

The time immediately before and after the meltdown is often not the best moment to discuss what is happening or has happened

At a later time, when everyone is feeling more settled, it might be helpful for the autistic person and their loved ones to talk about what would be helpful to do and say after a meltdown has happened

Some autistic people or their loved ones, may wish to forget about what has happened and carry on as normal (a meltdown does not have to be a big deal – if nobody was hurt for example – it may be better to just accept they are a part of your life together)

Others may want to talk about their experience in more depth

Some autistic people might get very angry and defensive if their loved ones try to talk to them about their recent meltdown, so learning how to communicate with one another is important...

...Finding the right time, using the right words, the right tone of voice, 'talking' in the right way (e.g. a text conversation might be more manageable than a verbal one)

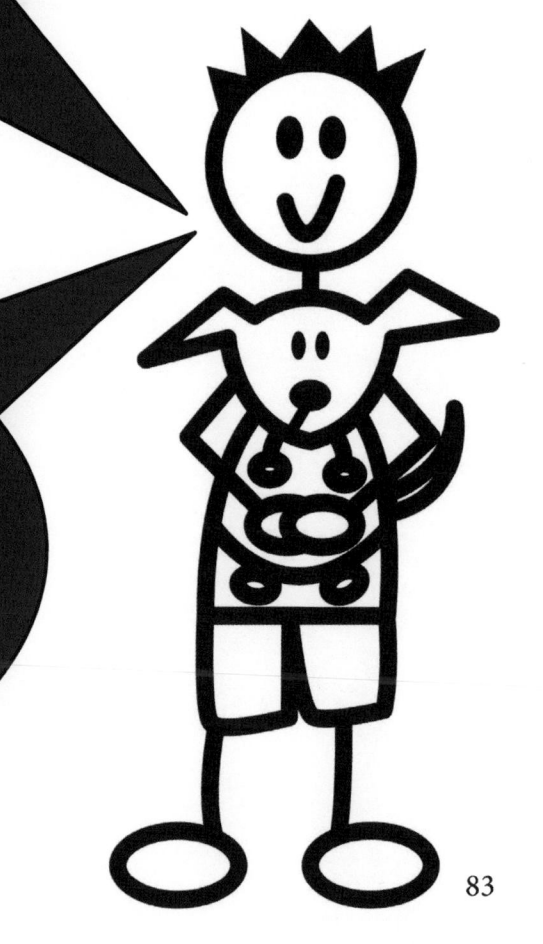

In order to help the autistic person deal with feelings of shame and embarrassment, reassurance that loved ones still see them as the same person, that things are OK and that nothing has changed can be really important to some autistic people

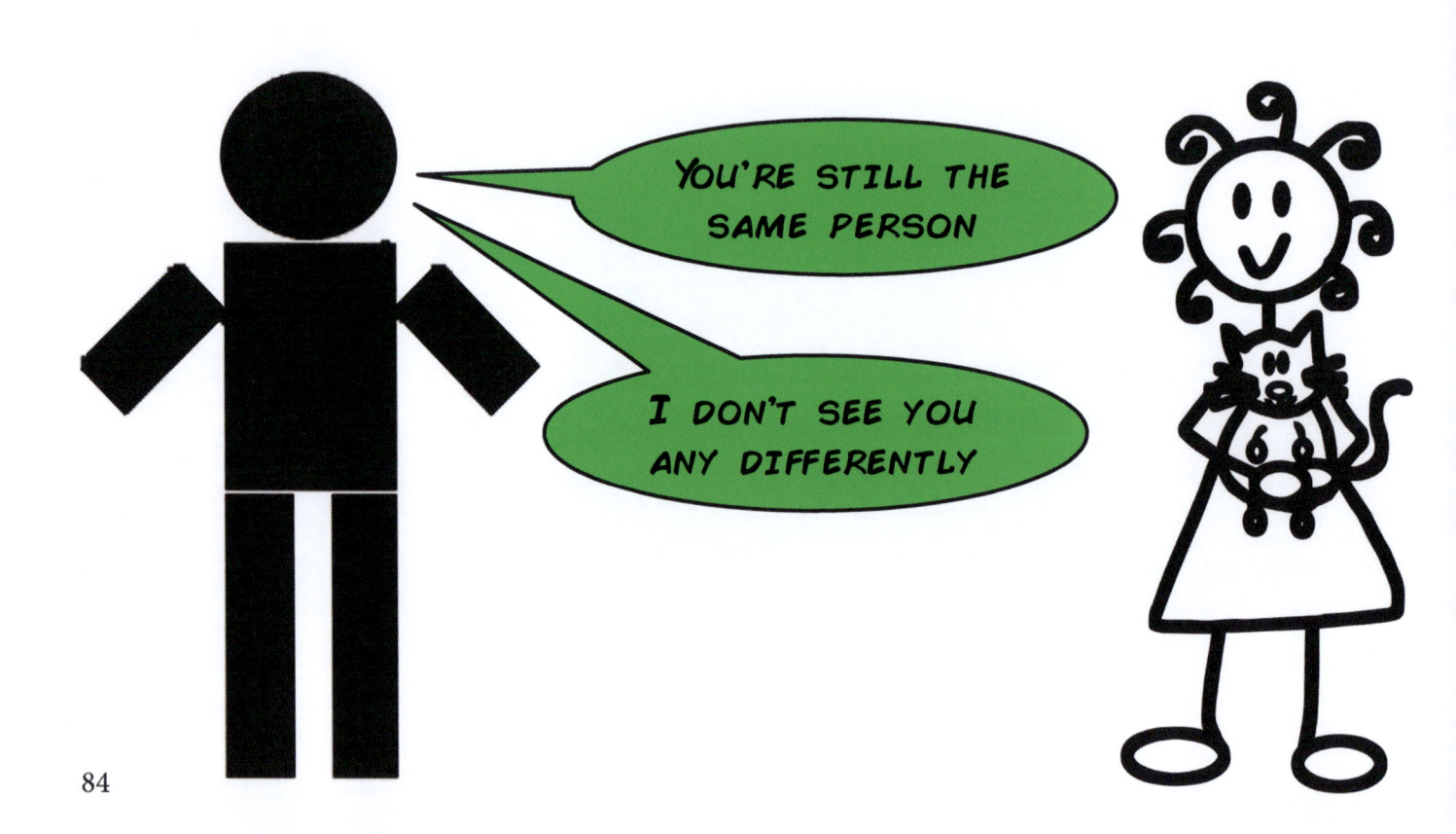

YOU'RE STILL THE SAME PERSON

I DON'T SEE YOU ANY DIFFERENTLY

Tips on how to talk to an autistic person about their meltdowns

- Don't get angry
- Show that you understand
- Use the word "we" rather than "you" as that might let them know you care and love them and that they are not alone
- Shift the focus to a positive e.g. "We have a problem, but we're going to find a solution for it"
- Texting or writing to each other might be better than having a verbal conversation
- Be mindful of when you try to have the conversation (not when they are tired or have had a busy day) and give them plenty of time
- If you know they have recently been trying really hard to just generally manage their behaviour, remain encouraging. Say something like "I know that you are very upset right now, but I know that you are also very good at calming yourself down" and "It feels like the end of the world right now but you will get over this. I know you can"
- Truly *hear* them when they tell you why it happened – because you can help get rid of this trigger next time

Here are some strategies that might help an autistic person recover after a meltdown and some suggestions on how loved ones could help:

Autistic people

- Be kind to yourself and look after yourself
- Consider rearranging your diary to allow you some time to recover
- Talk calmly about what happened with the people around you
- Reflect on why you think the meltdown happened and consider whether there were any prior signs or think about whether there was anything you could have done differently to prevent it
- Be aware that your behaviour might have been uncomfortable or upsetting to someone else. Listen to what they have to say and be considerate. They might want to talk about it
- Raise awareness of autism and meltdowns in your community
- In the long run, reassessing and rearranging your lifestyle to keep input levels down will be the best solution to managing meltdowns

Family members

- Try not to be judgmental or angry
- Educate yourself about meltdowns and understand that they are often out of the person's control
- Some autistic people feel embarrassed and want to be reassured that you still see them as the same person
- Give them some space or time alone to recover
- Be a team and try to work out together why the meltdown happened and how it might have been prevented
- Validate how the person feels by trying to put yourself in their shoes
- Ask them what they need from you – for example, do they need any help rearranging their diary? Do they want to talk about what happened? Ask them what you could have done that would have helped

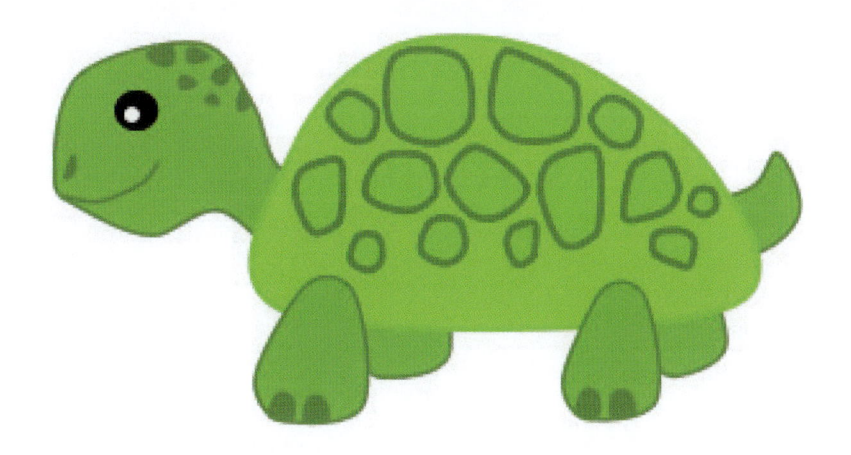

Shutdowns

Shutdowns are another reaction to too much input

Whereas a meltdown is more of an outward expression of feeling overstimulated, a shutdown is more of an inward one:

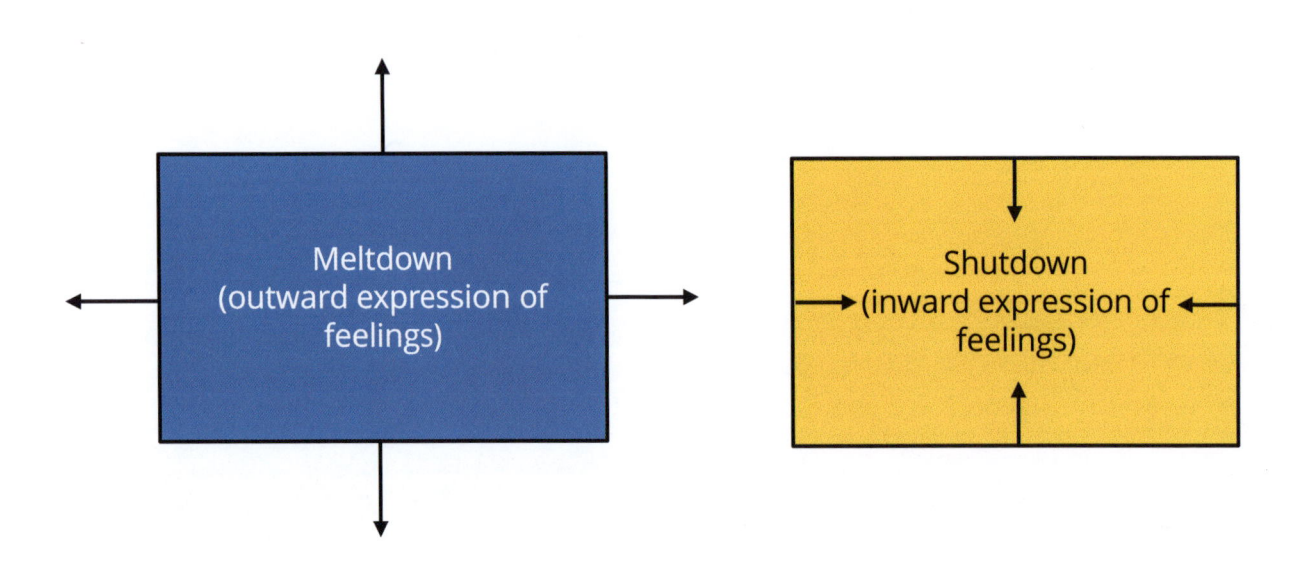

Meltdown (outward expression of feelings)

Shutdown (inward expression of feelings)

89

Shutdowns are a normal part of being autistic

Fortunately, for a lot of the time, a shutdown is a fleeting, brief experience and might last only a few minutes

An easy way for a neurotypical person to relate to this is to think about a time where you have felt very anxious and somebody asked you to say or do something, and you were unable to respond. You probably literally felt 'frozen' for a short moment

Other shutdowns are longer and might last several hours or even several days. These types of shutdown can be very debilitating and create limitations on how successfully an autistic person can lead their life. For example, a person who is in shutdown would not be able to go to work or to school

Other problems might be that the person won't eat, dress, bathe, participate in their hobbies, etc.

The consequence of being in shutdown can be sadness and very low mood:

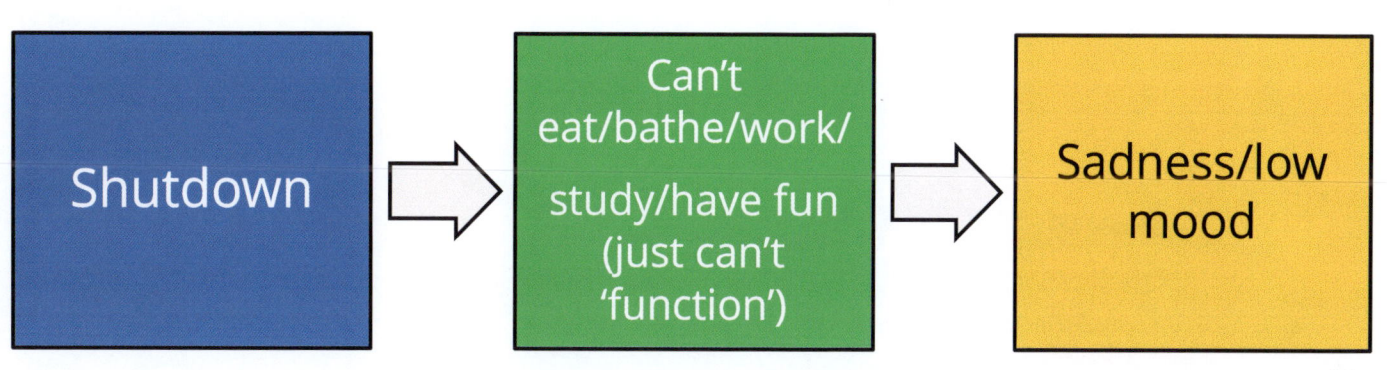

Shutdown → Can't eat/bathe/work/study/have fun (just can't 'function') → Sadness/low mood

Shutdowns as a coping mechanism

It might be helpful to think of shutdowns as a 'protection mechanism' - a shutting off of the brain so that it can't receive any more input

Shutdowns might be a way of regenerating more social energy (page 40). They might be a way of reducing the level of input in the bucket (page 24)

> I NEED TO SHUT DOWN IN ORDER TO RECOVER FOR THE NEXT DAY OR SITUATION

Shutdowns are sometimes very much needed. For many autistic people, they are helpful, soothing and restorative

Shutdowns are not because a person is stubborn or lazy. They are often involuntary

Be patient and compassionate with yourself or with your loved one

How to recover after a shutdown

When an autistic person is recovering from a shutdown, perhaps it might be helpful if the focus was on conserving energy and making tasks as easy to do as possible

It might be helpful to stop putting pressure on themselves to do activities that are 'non-essential' - now is the time to focus on only what is essential and doing the things that they find enjoyable

Hobbies can be a really good way to help someone emerge from their shutdown, even if the hobby needs to be adapted slightly to account for the person's loss of energy

The thing to remember is that shutdowns are often about a lack of energy... so you can help yourself or help your autistic loved one by reducing the amount of energy they need to use for various activities

Here are some strategies on how normal everyday tasks could be made easier for an autistic person who is in a shutdown:

Helping someone who won't eat	
How to help yourself:	**How to help your loved one:**
• Prepare for shutdowns in advance and have meals ready and available in the fridge or in the freezer • Have foods available that are literally easy to eat, such as liquids or soft foods	• Make and bring to them their favourite or 'normal' food • Stick to their regular eating times • Consider foods that are literally easy to eat, such as liquids or soft foods

Helping someone who won't bathe	
How to help yourself:	**How to help your loved one:**
Find alternative ways to maintain hygiene that use less energy such as dry shampoo, keeping hair always short so it's easier to manage long-term	• Run them a bath • Put out the bath mat and towel • Have their clothes ready for them when they have finished • Offer to wash or comb their hair

| **Helping someone who won't talk** ||
How to help yourself:	How to help your loved one:
Find alternative ways to communicate such as through writing, drawing or texting	- Reduce your eye contact - Keep language simple and concise, use short sentences - Ask questions that only require brief or one-word answers - Write/draw/text instead

All of these things can be made easier if the autistic person is happier and has more energy... so one awesome way to do that is to suggest that they attempt to have a go at their special interests or hobbies:

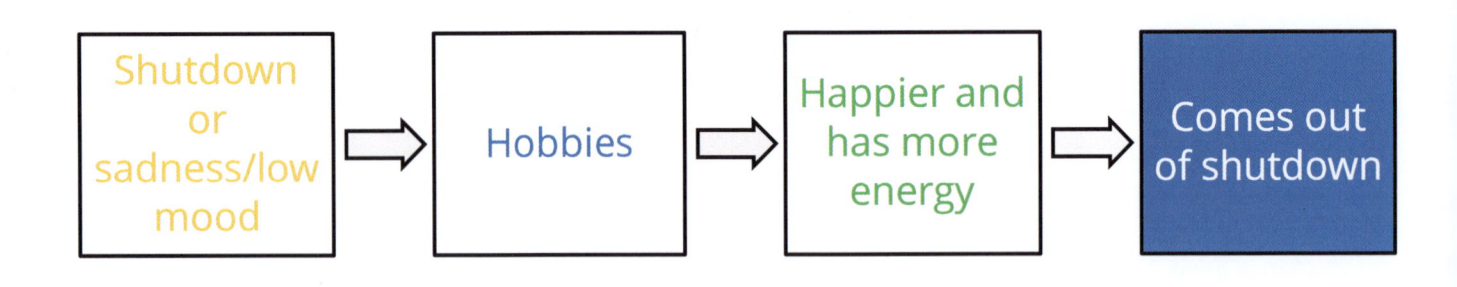

| Shutdown or sadness/low mood | → | Hobbies | → | Happier and has more energy | → | Comes out of shutdown |

Helping someone participate in hobbies	
How to help yourself:	How to help your loved one:
Find alternative ways to pursue hobby, e.g. may not be able to go out but could participate at home or read about it instead	• Adapt their hobby so that it can be done at home or from their bedroom • Talk to them about their hobby • Try participating in their hobby with them

Helping to prevent meltdowns and shutdowns

Preventing a meltdown is always better than having to experience one

The best way to manage a meltdown is to reduce the likelihood of one happening in the first place

This means an autistic person must know themselves well enough to know what their needs and their triggers are

It means having the skills and insight to arrange their lifestyle to reduce exposure to those triggers and ensure their needs are met

Trigger	How to manage it
Too much socialising	Ensure plenty of Alone Time, see people for only short durations of time, decline invitations as necessary, avoid going to public places during busy times
Too much sensory input	Reduce time spent in busy or noisy places, wear noise-reducing earplugs when out, put hood up to reduce peripheral vision, wear dark glasses, go out during quiet times of the day
Too little sensory input	Have something to fidget with, sit or sleep with a weighted blanket, get up and move about frequently
A feeling of having too much to do	This is probably a more complicated issue to resolve. It might be best to sit down with a loved one who will help you to organise yourself and your daily tasks

An autistic person might find it helpful to understand the technique of being able to say "no" to people or gaining the confidence to ask for adaptations to any situation that they find uncomfortable

Sometimes they'll be lucky and find someone who already knows the adaptations they need to make!

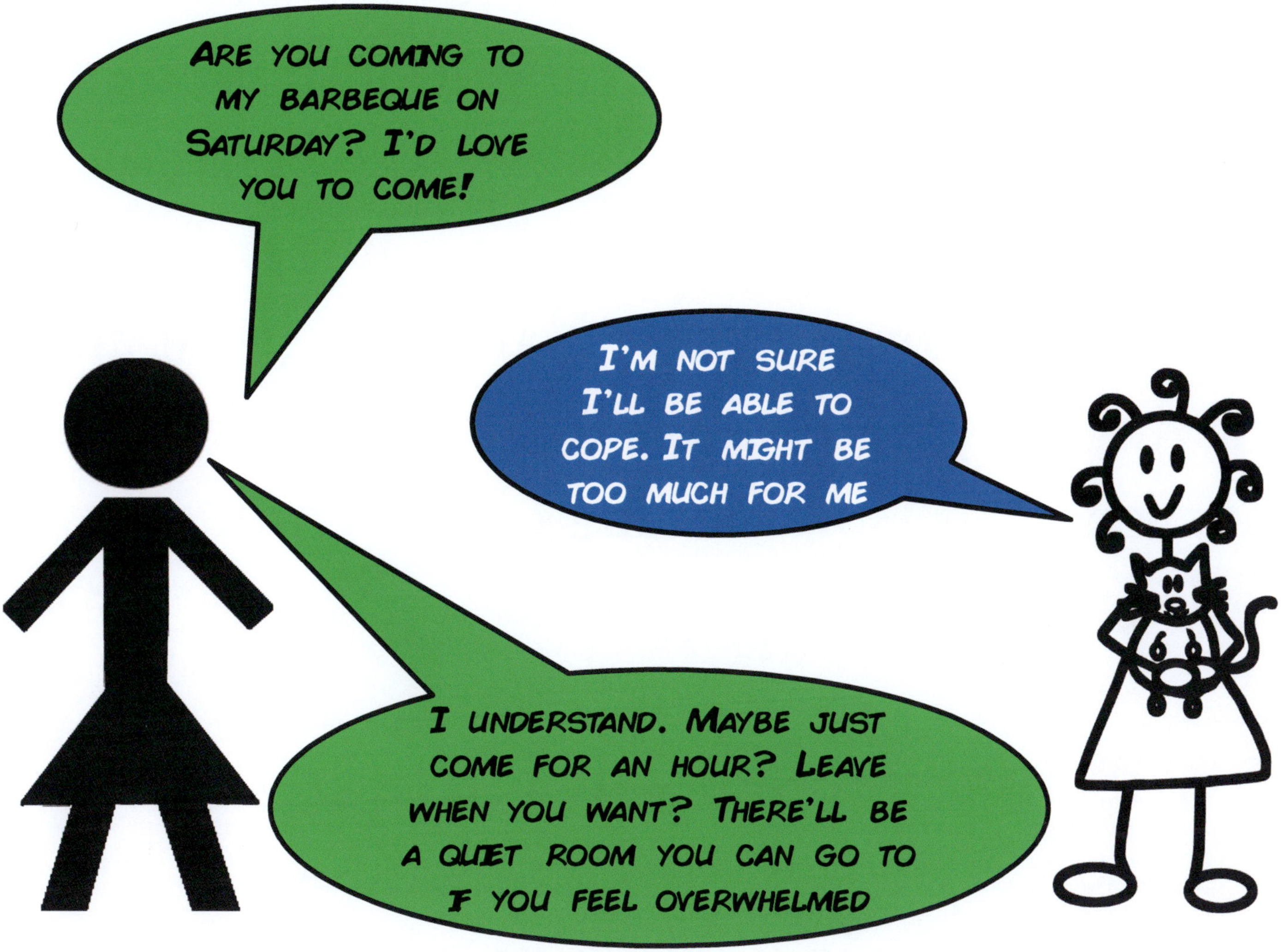
ARE YOU COMING TO MY BARBEQUE ON SATURDAY? I'D LOVE YOU TO COME!
I'M NOT SURE I'LL BE ABLE TO COPE. IT MIGHT BE TOO MUCH FOR ME
I UNDERSTAND. MAYBE JUST COME FOR AN HOUR? LEAVE WHEN YOU WANT? THERE'LL BE A QUIET ROOM YOU CAN GO TO IF YOU FEEL OVERWHELMED

In the long term, the ideal way to help stop meltdowns and shutdowns* is to improve life circumstances so that they occur less often

This is all about taking care not to feel overloaded by correctly managing input and having lots of Recharge Time (appreciate that an autistic person is going to need more down time than the average neurotypical person)

All of these things will lead to an autistic person living a less overwhelming and less anxiety-provoking life

*Shutdowns can sometimes be restorative but they can still be disruptive to daily life and so some autistic people would rather not have them

Summary

Meltdowns and shutdowns usually occur because an autistic person feels overstimulated by 'input'

Input is incoming information and can be sensory, social, self-awareness or executive function

The best way to prevent meltdowns and shutdowns from happening is to try to manage the amount of input an autistic person is dealing with in day to day life

Autistic people can find strategies they can use themselves to reduce this input, such as wearing earplugs in noisy environments or leaving social occasions a little earlier

Always remember to use each meltdown and shutdown as a learning point. Reflect on why they happened and consider what could have been done differently for a different outcome

Don't always see shutdowns as a negative - they might be a protective mechanism to help an autistic person stop receiving so much input

Many thanks for reading

Other books in The Visual Guides series at the time of writing:

Asperger's Syndrome
Asperger's Syndrome in 5-8 Year Olds
Asperger's Syndrome in 8-11 Year Olds
Asperger's Syndrome in 12-16 Year Old Girls
Asperger's Syndrome and Further Education
Asperger's Syndrome (for ASD/NT Couples)
Asperger's Syndrome: Socialising & Social Energy
Asperger's Syndrome and Anxiety
Asperger's Syndrome: Helping Siblings
Asperger's Syndrome and Puberty
Adapting Therapy for People on the Autism Spectrum
Asperger's Syndrome and Emotions
Asperger's Syndrome and Communication
Asperger's Syndrome and Executive Function
Asperger's Syndrome: Understanding Challenging Behaviour
Asperger's Syndrome and Eating Habits

New titles are continually being produced so keep an eye out!

Printed in Great Britain
by Amazon